Basic and Clinical Science of Substance Related Disorders

Bibliotheca Psychiatrica

No. 168

Series Editor   *Bernd Saletu*, Vienna

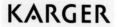 Basel · Freiburg · Paris · London · New York ·
New Delhi · Bangkok · Singapore · Tokyo · Sydney

Symposium 'Basic and Clinical Science of Substance Related Disorders',
Basel, May 20, 1998

....

Basic and Clinical Science of Substance Related Disorders

Volume Editor   *Dieter Ladewig*, Basel

13 figures and 8 tables, 1999

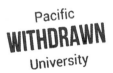

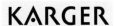

KARGER   Basel · Freiburg · Paris · London · New York ·
New Delhi · Bangkok · Singapore · Tokyo · Sydney

··························
Dieter Ladewig

Department of Psychiatry
University of Basel
Basel (Switzerland)

Library of Congress Cataloging-in-Publication Data
Basic and clinical science of substance related disorders / volume editor, D. Ladewig.
(Bibliotheca psychiatrica; no. 168)
Includes bibliographical references and indexes.
1. Substance abuse. 2. Substance abuse – Epidemiology. I. Ladewig, Dieter, 1938– . II. Series.
[DNLM: 1. Substance-Related Disorders – epidemiology. W1 BI429 no. 168 1999]
RC564.B3635 1999 616.86–dc21
ISBN 3–8055–6870–3 (hardcover : alk. paper)
ISSN 0067–8147

Bibliographic Indices. This publication is listed in bibliographic services, including Current Contents® and Index Medicus.

©Copyright 1999 by S. Karger AG, P.O. Box, CH–4009 Basel (Switzerland)
www.karger.com
Printed in Switzerland on acid-free paper by Reinhardt Druck, Basel
ISBN 3–8055–6870–3

Contents

VII Editor's Foreword
Ladewig, D. (Basel)

VIII Preface
Müller-Spahn, F. (Basel)

Biology

1 The Hypothalamic-Pituitary-Adrenocortical System: A Biological Substrate of Vulnerability to Drug Addiction
Spanagel, R. (Munich)

Epidemiology

7 Early Developmental Stages of Substance Abuse and Dependence. Examples from a Prospective Longitudinal Study
Wittchen, H.-U.; Lieb, R.; Perkonigg, A. (Munich)

Clinical Science

23 Aspects of the Psychosocial Consequences and Biological Evaluation of Heroin Treatments
Stohler, R. (Zürich)

29 Comorbidity Research in Substance Use Disorders
Preisig, M. (Lausanne); Fenton, B.T. (Geneva)

40 From Neuroscience to Psychoscience. The Integration of Drug Therapy and Psychotherapy into a Coordinated Dependency Management Project
Besson, J. (Lausanne)

45   **Randomized Open Efficacy Study of Naltrexone vs. Acamprosate vs. Disulfiram Combined with Cognitive-Behavioral Psychotherapy in Preventing Alcohol Relapse**
Bardeleben, U. von; Knoch, H.; Biedert, E.; Ihde, T.; Ladewig, D. (Basel)

49   **Clinical Addiction Research between Health Care Responsibility and Basic Research**
Ladewig, D. (Basel)

Historical

56   **Alcoholism Today.** The Rebirth of Ideologies of Individual Blame
Müller, R. (Lausanne)

64   **Author Index**
65   **Subject Index**

....
Editor's Foreword

This symposium took place on May 20, 1998 at the Department of Psychiatry of Basel University and brought together scientists from various disciplines. It was designed to give the attending clinicians an insight into the diversity of modern addiction research. The symposium and the subsequent publication of the proceedings were made possible by the generous support from the Freiwillige Akademische Gesellschaft Basel (an association set up to promote teaching and research at the University of Basel) and F. Hoffmann-La Roche AG. I should particularly like to thank the president of the Freiwillige Akademische Gesellschaft, Dr. Christoph Albrecht, and Dr. Wolfdieter Hetzel and Dr. Susan E. Hilton from Roche for their efficient help. Thanks are also due to my secretary, Sandra Zubler, for her highly constructive management of the manuscripts, the translation team at F. Hoffmann-La Roche AG for their extremely professional contributions and to the publisher S. Karger AG for their support in publishing this volume.

Prof. Dr. *D. Ladewig*

Preface

The Department of Psychiatry of the University of Basel can look back on a long tradition in the domain of addiction research. The social- and health-political importance of prevention, diagnostics and therapy of different addiction disorders was recognised very early. Here Basel has adopted a leading role, nationally and internationally. Indeed, only a few clinics have at their disposal such a specialised infrastructure in the area of withdrawal and maintenance treatment of drug dependence for both in- and out-patients. This would not have been possible without the efforts of Prof. Ladewig and his co-workers. Prof. Ladewig must indeed be seen as one of the pioneers of national and international addiction research.

This symposium was organised on the occasion of his 60th birthday and honours a scientist and clinician who has acquired high merits in this area. It deals with highly relevant topics in the domain of basic and clinical addiction research. Each psychiatric disorder has a biological, psychological and social dimension. The organisers have succeeded in winning speakers with an international reputation. They will present some of their latest findings concerning these various aspects.

Prof. Dr. *F. Müller-Spahn*

Ladewig D (ed): Basic and Clinical Science of Substance Related Disorders.
Bibl Psychiatr. Basel, Karger, 1999, No 168, pp 1–6

....

The Hypothalamic-Pituitary-Adrenocortical System: A Biological Substrate of Vulnerability to Drug Addiction

Rainer Spanagel

Max Planck Institute of Psychiatry, University of Munich, Germany

The time to onset of compulsive drug-seeking behaviour varies with the drug of abuse. While intravenous heroin use, for example, is rapidly addicting, it may be years before an alcohol drinker manifests addictive behaviour. Chronic alcohol consumption can be broken down into three phases, beginning with the initiation or acquisition of drinking behaviour and progressing to controlled and, in some cases, ultimately to uncontrolled drinking. One of the major questions about the aetiology of drug addiction is why some individuals become addicted while others do not. In fact, humans show enormous individual differences in their drug-taking behaviour. Many people have tried drugs at least once, but only a few persist in using them and develop addictive behaviour. For the others, drug use remains at most an occasional recreational activity. Individual vulnerability to the effects of drugs of abuse is determined by numerous factors, the most important being genetic predisposition, pharmacological prehistory, social context and stress. Additionally, it is assumed that drugs require special biologically vulnerable systems to develop their abuse potential. Little is known about the biological substrates involved in mediating individual sensitivity to drugs of abuse, but recent studies indicate that the hypothalamic-pituitary-adrenocortical (HPA) system and endogenous opioid systems play a crucial role.

Results from animal studies suggest that stressful experiences increase the vulnerability to drug self-administration. Similarly, plasma levels of corticosterone influence the psychomotor stimulant and reinforcing effects of various drugs of abuse. Work in our laboratory has shown that adrenalectomy drastically alters ethanol drinking behaviour in rats. In a four-bottle free-choice paradigm between water, 5%, 10% and 20% (v/v) ethanol, ethanol intake in sham-operated animals averaged 5–6 g/kg/day during the 1st week of exposure, as compared with 2–3 g/kg/day for the adrenalectomised rats. Replacement of corticosterone with slow-release corticosterone pellets almost normalised ethanol intake in the adrenalectomised group. In subsequent experiments we measured ethanol consumption during relapse. Daily ethanol intake was seen to stabilise over several weeks of voluntary consumption. A 2-week period of ethanol deprivation was followed, however, by a transient increase in consumption, with ethanol intake increasing for several days to nearly twice the baseline levels. This deprivation effect resembles an incentive motivation for ethanol. Interestingly, adrenalectomised animals did not display a deprivation effect, although corticosterone replacement in these animals led to the same level of ethanol intake observed in sham-operated rats. These simple manipulations show that circulating corticosterone levels and HPA activity can profoundly influence the initiation and recurrence of drug-seeking behaviour.

HPA activity is regulated by glucocorticoid receptors (GRs). In particular, GRs are responsible for the negative feedback effects of corticosterone on HPA activity. Activation of the HPA system is driven mainly by hypothalamic corticotropin-releasing hormone (CRH) and vasopressin. These secretagogues, which are produced in either the same or distinct neurons of the paraventricular nucleus, act synergistically to enhance the release of pituitary pro-opiomelano-cortin-derived peptides (ACTH and endorphins). Adrenal glucocorticoid hormone secretion (corticosterone in rodents, cortisol in humans) is subsequently stimulated mainly by ACTH. Certain hormonal responses to external stimuli such as stress cannot be adequately controlled by the hypothalamus alone, and effective regulation is dependent on extrahypothalamic integration. Extrahypo-thalamic integration of HPA activity is provided mainly by noradrenergic innervation, the amygdala and the hippocampus. In general, the hippocampus inhibits HPA activity, while the action of the amygdala is mainly permissive. In the hippocampus GRs are responsible for the negative feedback of adrenal steroids on HPA activity.

Effects of Morphine in Transgenic Mice with Impaired GR function

The involvement of GRs in sensitivity to the effects of drugs of abuse was studied in transgenic mice with impaired GR function. These mice bear a type II GR antisense construct under the control of a neurofilament promoter. Insertion of an antisense RNA-generating transgene produces an animal with defective glucocorticoid feedback. It should be mentioned that complete GR knockouts are not viable; GR-deficient mice die of respiratory failure within a few hours of birth. Mice bearing the aforementioned antisense construct are viable, however, and develop normally despite impaired GR function. We tested the psychomotor stimulant effects of the prototypic opioid agonist morphine in these animals. Animals were subjected to an open-field test following injection of saline or morphine. Transgenic mice exhibited a stronger locomotor-activating response to morphine than did appropriate controls. This response was dose-dependent. Significantly, basal activity and locomotor activity following saline injections did not differ between transgenic mice and controls.

The psychomotor-activating effects of morphine and other drugs of abuse are associated with increased dopamine release in the mesolimbic system. This system consists of A10 dopaminergic neurons, which arise in the ventral tegmental area and project mainly to the nucleus accumbens and prefrontal cortex. The nucleus accumbens can be seen as the interface for motivation and goal-directed behaviour. In other words, dopamine release in this nucleus seems to be linked to reinforcement processes and motor-activating effects. In more recent studies we have addressed the question of whether transgenic mice with impaired GR function exhibit altered basal and morphine-induced dopamine release in the nucleus accumbens. For this purpose we used the novel approach of in vivo microdialysis in freely moving mice. Although basal dopamine levels did not differ between transgenic and control mice, administration of morphine (15 mg/kg i.p.) to drug-naive animals enhanced dopamine release significantly in transgenic mice but only slightly in controls. It should be noted that mesolimbic A10 dopamine neurons express GRs, and that GRs modulate dopamine release in a state-dependent manner. Corticosterone levels were also determined in the same microdialysis samples. Mean basal intracerebral levels of corticosterone were enhanced in transgenic mice as compared with naive controls. Morphine produced an increase in both transgenic mice and controls, but corticosterone levels were higher in the transgenic animals at all measurement times. Consistent with the hypothesis that individual vulnerability to drug-seeking behaviour is determined by HPA activity, the present results show that mice with impaired GR function, and thus elevated intracerebral corticosterone levels, are more sensitive than controls to the unconditioned behavioural effects of morphine and exhibit augmented dopamine release.

We also investigated the behaviour of transgenic mice when offered access to morphine in a free-choice paradigm. In the 1st week transgenic mice self-administered significantly more morphine than controls, but by the end of week 2 self-administration rates had become similar. These findings indicate that GRs are also important factors in susceptibility to the reinforcing effects of morphine, and that the initiation of drug-taking behaviour is at least partly controlled by GRs and subsequent HPA activity. It remains to be determined whether these receptors play an essential role in relapse behaviour in drug-seeking animals. In conclusion, one may reasonably speculate that genetic vulnerability to the effects of drugs of abuse is influenced by altered GR levels or by dysfunction of these receptors.

Pharmacological manipulation of corticosterone secretion or HPA activity has been mooted as a potentially valuable new approach to treating drug abuse. We therefore tested the possibility of influencing a genetic predisposition determined by impaired GRs. Long-term treatment with antidepressants is known to influence the expression of GRs. In our experiment transgenic mice were given moclobemide (15 mg/kg/day) for 8 weeks in their drinking water. Moclobemide is a highly selective and reversible monoamine oxidase A inhibitor. Prolonged moclobemide treatment 'normalised' unconditioned psychomotor stimulant responses to morphine injection in transgenic mice to those seen in controls. It is important to note that antidepressant treatment did not alter morphine-induced locomotion in control animals. Corticosterone levels were also normalised in the transgenic animals treated with moclobemide, and enhanced, morphine-induced dopamine release decreased. In the control animals, prolonged administration of moclobemide had no effect on morphine-induced dopamine release. In pretreated transgenic animals, by contrast, the same dose of morphine had a diminished stimulatory effect on mesolimbic dopamine release.

Prolonged antidepressant treatment thus seems to normalise HPA system activity. This leads to 'normal' responses to the unconditioned effects of morphine. Moreover, the neurochemical events which mediate these unconditioned effects do not deviate from the 'norm' following antidepressant treatment. It is hoped that these results will open up new approaches to preventing drug abuse. It might be feasible, for example, to identify genetically predisposed individuals by neuroendocrine challenge tests and then institute long-term antidepressant therapy to reduce their vulnerability to drug abuse.

Ethanol Exposure and Withdrawal in CRH-R1-Deficient Mice

As mentioned before, hypothalamic CRH and its two receptors, CRH-R1 and CRH-R2, are the main driving force in activation of the HPA system. CRH-R1 is highly expressed in the anterior pituitary, neocortex, hippocampus, amygdala and cerebellum and functions as the prime mediator in stress-induced HPA system activation by triggering the immediate release of ACTH from the anterior pituitary. Encouraged by our findings with GR-impaired transgenic mice, we hypothesised that alterations in CRH receptor signalling might influence vulnerability to drugs of abuse.

Very recently a CRH-R1-deficient mouse has been created using homologous recombination to delete the G-protein coupling domain in embryonic stem cells. In the absence of a G-protein coupling domain, activation of second messenger systems and transmission of ligand-induced signals are impossible. Morphological analysis of these mutant mice revealed major alterations. Marked accumulation of CRH peptide was seen by immunohistochemistry in discrete areas of the brain, including the hypothalamic paraventricular nucleus, amygdala, hippocampus and cerebral cortex. Histological analysis of the adrenal glands did not reveal any apparent changes in the adrenal cortex, including the zona fasciculata, which is the major site of corticosterone production; but the diameter of the adrenal medulla was reduced by 50% in homozygous mutants. The importance of CRH-R1 in regulating HPA system activity, particularly during stress, is highlighted by the fact that only very low post-stress corticosterone levels are detected in CRH-R1-deficient mice, whereas wild types show a 10-fold increase in corticosterone release following swim stress.

According to the opponent process theory of motivation, withdrawal is the major driving force in drug-seeking behaviour. In the case of ethanol, it is primarily anxiety-related behaviour during withdrawal which triggers further drinking. We tested anxiety-related behaviour during ethanol withdrawal in CRH-R1-deficient mice using an anxiety test battery, which included a light dark box test in which transitions and time spent in a brightly lit compartment were measured. Mice were subjected to forced ethanol drinking procedure and then tested under withdrawal conditions. All mice exhibited signs of withdrawal, including increased latency to enter the brightly lit compartment. Comparisons of light avoidance behaviour by genotype revealed significant differences under basal versus withdrawal conditions for wild types and heterozygous mutants, but not for homozygous mutants. Furthermore, during withdrawal CRH-R1-deficient animals showed shorter latencies to enter the lit compartment than wild-type mice, entered it more frequently and stayed there longer. The performance parameters for heterozygous mutants were between those for homozygous and wild-type animals for all tests under withdrawal conditions, suggesting a gene dosage effect of CRH-R1. These findings show that the CRH-R1 receptor – along with others such as the NMDA and GABA$_A$ receptors – contributes to mediating the anxiety-related behaviour observed under ethanol withdrawal conditions.

Conclusion

It has been postulated that stress, HPA system activity and glucocorticoids are organised in a pathophysiological chain determining vulnerability to drug effects and drug abuse. As indicated in the present paper, transgenic mice with impaired GR function and CRH-R1 knockouts appear to be excellent animal models for further elucidating the causal relationship between HPA system activity and sensitivity to the acute effects and addictive properties of drugs of abuse. It is clear, however, that the HPA system cannot be the sole biological substrate of vulnerability to drugs of abuse. Among other things, alterations in endogenous opioid systems also seem to be of particular importance in determining sensitivity to drug effects relevant to the induction and maintenance of addictive behaviour.

PD Dr. R. Spanagel, Max-Planck-Institut für Psychiatrie,
Kraepelinstrasse 2, D–80804 München (Germany)
Tel. +49 89 30622–288, Fax +49 89 30622–569, E-Mail spanagel@mpipsykl.mpg.de

Ladewig D (ed): Basic and Clinical Science of Substance Related Disorders.
Bibl Psychiatr. Basel, Karger, 1999, No 168, pp 7–22

····················

Early Developmental Stages of Substance Abuse and Dependence

Examples from a Prospective Longitudinal Study

Hans-Ulrich Wittchen, Roselind Lieb, Axel Perkonigg

Max Planck Institute of Psychiatry, Clinical Psychiatry and Epidemiology Unit, Munich, Germany

Despite much recent research [1–24], the etiopathogenesis of drug abuse and dependence remains uneludicated. The explanatory models offered to date are similar in that all are multifactorial, albeit of variable complexity, and involve interaction between individual vulnerability, the environment, and risk factors. However, they differ in the importance they ascribe to genetics, neurobiology, psychology and the psychosocial dimension. In particular, there has been no systematic study characterizing the nature, strength and chronology of factor interaction across all substance classes, use stages, and user subgroups defined by age, sex and risk. This makes it difficult to develop rational strategies for prevention and therapeutic intervention.

In an attempt to fill these gaps, a focus of current addiction research is the design of improved and applicable longitudinal models, e.g. based cohort studies at critical life and development stages. Most of these models follow the current classification of substance use disorders in ICD-10 [25] and DSM-IV [26] by concentrating on substance-specific vulnerabilities, risks and consequences at the onset and in the progression of abuse and dependence. However, a number of methodological challenges arise, a few of which will be highlighted below.

Approaches

Sampling

There are a number of possible approaches in devising such longitudinal studies. Commonest, because practicable and cheap, is the 'sample of convenience' comprising subjects already in contact with a specialist unit for an addiction problem. Retrospective questioning is used to reconstruct the addiction onset and development history, supplemented on occasion by information from family or peer group members. This approach carries obvious inferential pitfalls. First, the findings depend strongly on the subject's retrospective reconstruction of events, his current level of distress, and intervention-induced attributions. Second, negative pognostic indicators, especially those for onset, are systematically overestimated in subjects who have already come to clinical attention; protective factors on the other hand are correspondingly underestimated. Similar, if lesser, dangers apply to the second common addiction strategy, namely preemptive recruitment of help-seekers, e.g. through newspaper advertisements or initial contacts at counselling centers. Studies in at-risk and high-risk subjects are midway between patient studies and epidemiological surveys in the general population. They can be a highly efficient and informative strategy, especially when performed prospectively. Nevertheless, they presuppose valid and representative sampling and sample definition in defining risk and high risk.

Design

The ideal framework for investigating etiopathogenesis in development terms is the representative population study with a prospective longitudinal design. Such studies are complex, expensive and time-consuming. They also have the drawback of relative inefficiency, particularly if the addictive behavior in question is anticipated in only a small subsample. This often results in relatively small sample sizes for specific target groups, e.g. opiate users, despite impressively large total numbers. Such strategies are therefore often combined with representative cohort studies. In a two-stage design, the risk group of interest is identified by screening before proceeding to a more in-depth clinical study interview. Representative population studies are further complicated by much more laborious analyses, often requiring weighting procedures, depending on the type of sampling plan. As these are not built in to standard statistical packages, sometimes requiring highly difficult interactive programs instead, it is often a time-consuming challenge to describe even such simple parameters as prevalence and incidence. A further drawback of representative population studies is that they rely on standardized survey instruments that often lack the clinical subtlety required by clinically oriented investigators. Reviews of current etiological studies in substance use disorders [12] have highlighted the major deficit represented by the continued predominance of retrospective studies, which are of limited predictive value whether in clinical or patient populations. Clinical early-stage studies remain extraordinarily rare, prompting recent decisions of federal funding agencies in the US and Germany to earmark resources to correct the imbalance.

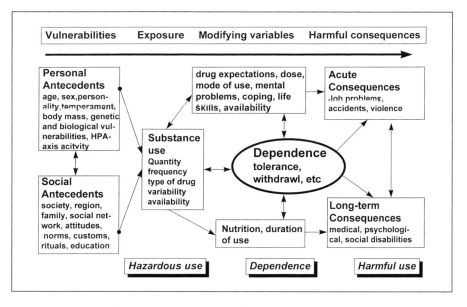

Fig. 1. EDSP: Conceptual framework of risks.

Assessment Instruments

Despite a general trend towards convergence, the assessment methods used in diagnosis (e.g. definition and quantification of dependence characteristics) and use characterization (amount and frequency) vary widely in many addiction studies. This creates extraordinary difficulties for the meta-analyses of different data sets which could be highly desirable for increasing statistical power. An important deficit of research to date is that only a few assessment and modeling studies consider the substance interactions and comorbidity patterns which can obviously be crucial not only in initiating regular use but in shaping the development and course of dependence.

Modeling Theory and Methods in the Early Developmental Stages of Psychopathology Study

Modeling Theory

The Early Developmental Stages of Psychopathology (EDSP) study is based on the generic model for the development of substance use disorders shown in figure 1. This model itself derives from the concept of abuse and dependence on psychotropic substances operationalized in DSM-IV [26] and with minor differences in ICD-10 [25]. Its key elements are the development

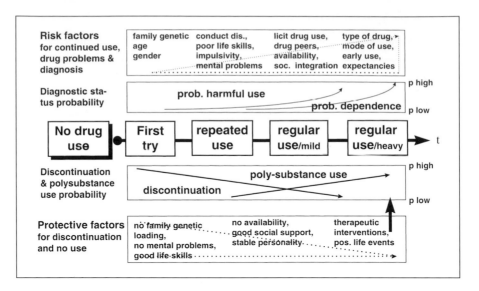

Fig. 2. Conceptual framework for transition analyses.

of harmful use, which replaces the old abuse concept, and the dependence syndrome, which is described in substance-specific terms. The dimensionally structured dependence syndrome is distinguished in content and conception from the more socially oriented criteria of harmful use, which need no longer automatically be a preliminary stage of dependence.

This model provides the design framework shown in figure 2 for investigating the probabilities of transition at various stages of substance use and in a similar way (not shown) for the development of substance use disorders. This distinguishes both substance-specific modes of behavior – which can be broadly differentiated as 'first exposure', 'repeated use' and the transitions to 'regular light' and 'regular heavy' use – and risk and protective factors, which, depending on substance use stage, use behavior and substance abused, can have varying effects on the probability of harmful use, dependence development, polysubstance abuse and use cessation.

Design and Aims

Sponsored by the German government's Biological and Psychosocial Factors of Drug Abuse research program, in 1995 we launched a prospective epidemiological longitudinal study of complex design to investigate a representative sample of 3,021 14- to 24-year-olds from the greater Munich area.

The study is divided into three waves (fig. 3), the first conducted in 1995, the second in 1996/7 and the last currently being completed in 1998/9.

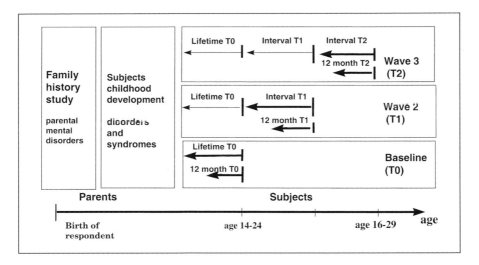

Fig. 3. EDSP design and diagnostic information.

A special feature is its direct link to a family study, as well as to various supplementary studies – including population lab experiments – in which at-risk study subjects are recalled to test certain etiological hypotheses (such as those based on stress or anxiety). The family history study (left column) provides information of parental substance use as well as mental disorders and on the subject's development (birth or early childhood, school and health development) shown in the second column. On the right are shown the three study waves, in each of which lifetime, interval and 12-month data were collected on symptoms, use pattern, use and diagnoses.

The general goal of the EDSP is to establish: (1) how often use, abuse and dependence occur in 14- to 24-year-olds; (2) how often 'one-time', 'regular' and 'harmful' use and dependence syndromes develop, and (3) what factors determine these stage changes. In addition, we are especially interested in the stability of use and disorder patterns in this age-group, as well as in spontaneous cessation and its determinants.

Method

As the methods, design and results were recently described in detail in a special issue of *European Addiction Research* 1998 [28–32, see also ref. 33–35] only brief information will be given here. The study was conducted by clinically trained investigators, mainly graduate psychologists, who personally interviewed subjects and their parents using a lengthy (2-hour) standardized diagnostic instrument (Munich-Composite International Diagnostic Interview) [36], supplemented by a variety of questionnaires and specific interview sections dealing with psychosocial factors, documentation of risk and vulnerability factors, and consequences and

Table 1. Prevalence of substance-specific consumption patterns in 14- to 24-year-olds

Substance class	Pattern of use			
	once	repeated	regular	total
Cannabis	6.5	11.0	15.5	33.0
Amphetamines (Ecstasy)	1.0	1.5	2.4	5.0
Sedatives	0.2	0.7	0.7	1.6
Opiates	0.8	1.1	1.5	3.4
Cocaine	1.4	1.4	1.2	4.0
Hallucinogens	1.1	0.7	1.4	3.2

Other substances (inhalants) total 2.3%.

implications of use. A major feature was that application of the instrument in the different study waves was designed to monitor susceptibilities, risks, use patterns, time courses and use motivation as closely as possibly over time and relate them to changes in risk and protective factors for vulnerability. The aims of the family history study were not only to identify familial risks, such as availability of legal and illegal substances in the household, but also to investigate use and dependence patterns and parental use behavior, thereby examining family genetics in the broadest sense [37–39].

Findings

Results of EDSP Baseline Study (1994/95)

Table 1 shows the frequency (weighted prevalence) of psychotropic substance use in 14- to 24-year-olds from the baseline investigation. The figures are percentages weighted by the individual's representation in terms of age and gender in the total population, corrected for nonresponse and systematic dropouts [see also ref. 40]. As expected, the most commonly mentiond substance was cannabis, which 33% of all 14- to 24-year-olds had used at least once in their life. In second place were amphetamines and especially Ecstasy, followed by cocaine, hallucinogens and opiates, a noteworthy point in the latter case being the high proportion of regular codeine users, a characteristic feature of the Munich situation. Sedative use was relatively low, at 1.6%. In terms of use pattern, regular users (defined as ever use at least 5 times) predominated, while the proportion of one-time users was lowest with cannabis. Other substances (e.g. inhalants) were mentioned with a prevalence of 2.3%.

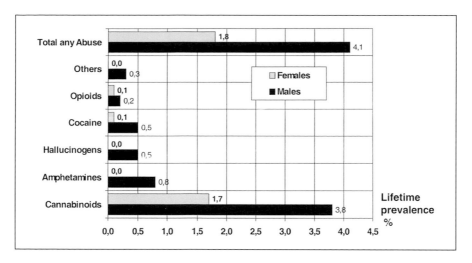

Fig. 4. EDSP: Lifetime prevalence of DSM-IV abuse in 14- to 24-year-olds in 1995 (baseline).

Figure 4 shows that – based on DMS-IV abuse criteria – 4.1% of all male subjects and 1.8% of all female subjects had already developed a manifest abuse pattern, most commonly of the cannabis type, followed by amphetamines and hallucinogens. If we incorporate the exposure rates from table 1, we find a particularly high abuse diagnosis risk in the case of stimulants (5:1) and hallucinogens (6:1) by comparison with cannabis (11:1).

A clinically manifest dependence syndrome, as defined by DSM-IV criteria, was identified in 2.5% of males and 1.6% of females in our study (fig. 5). Here again, cannabis dependence predominated, followed primarily by stimulants. Comparison of the exposure rate with the risk of developing a dependence problem again showed a maximum for hallucinogens and stimulants (8:1 and 9:1, respectively) and opiates (cannabis as a reference: 15:1).

However, the proportion with a conspicuous use pattern was distinctly higher among lifetime ever users. Figure 6 describes – in addition to the manifest abuse and dependence patterns in figures 4 and 5 – the proportion of regular heavy users among lifetime ever users at baseline interview and the proportion of those who already had at least a subthreshold diagnosis [see also ref. 30]. At 50–70% of all users, the proportion of conspicuous use patterns was very high, especially in the hallucinogen user group. The high proportion of individuals with subthreshold diagnoses – i.e. a partial dependence syndrome – is particularly striking.

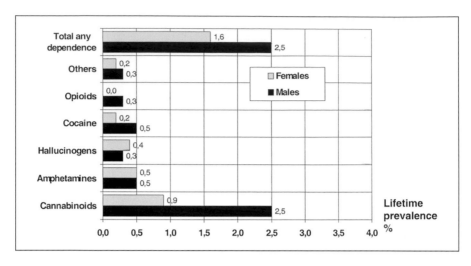

Fig. 5. Lifetime prevalence of DSM-IV dependence in 14- to 24-year-olds (EDSP, 1995 baseline).

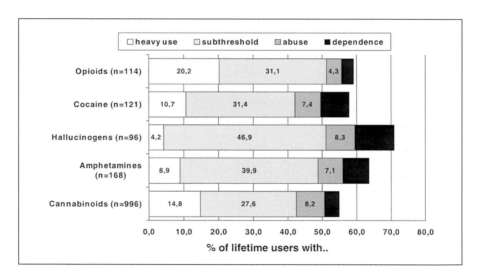

Fig. 6. Heavy use, subthreshold and threshold (abuse/dependence) disorders among lifetime drug users (EDSP, 1995).

Table 2 shows that there is a considerable overlap between substance classes in terms of diagnoses of abuse and dependence. This finding indicates a considerable comorbidity between various classes of substance use disorders. We found that 18% of the subjects with a cannabis-related substance use disorder also fulfill criteria for an amphethamine-related disorder, 4% for a

Table 2. Frequency (in %) of subjects with one-substance use disorders also meeting criteria for abuse or dependence of one or more other substance class

Among those with substance use disorder of ...	How many (%) also other substance disorders					
	cannabis	amphet-amines	halluci-nogens	cocaine	opiates	other
Cannabis	*80*	18	4	12	4	6
Amphetamines/Ecstasy	88	*0*	76	56	20	28
Hallucinogens	95	100	*0*	47	11	26
Cocaine	79	74	47	*21*	32	32
Opiates	56	56	22	67	*33*	44
Others	80	50	40	50	40	*20*

Weighted % because multiple disorder numbers sum up to more than 100%.

hallucinogen-related disorder, and 12% for abuse/dependence of cocaine. A relatively high proportion of cannabis users (80%) fulfill exclusively criteria for cannabis abuse/dependence. A quite different picture emerges with amphetamines, where we find not a single case fulfilling only criteria for amphetamine abuse/dependence. There is also marked overlap with hallucinogen-, cocaine- and opiate-related substance use disorders. Findings were almost identical for hallucinogens and the other substances. The first column with the high percentages for cannabis also suggests that, with the exception of opiates, almost all persons with substance use disorders from different substance classes also show abuse/dependence of cannabis.

In summary, the EDSP baseline study showed that a third of all 14- to 24-year-olds (males 40% and females 30%) have tried at least one psychotropic substance at least once. 17% of all 14- to 24-year-olds (males 20% and females 15%) are regular users. The dominant substance is cannabis, followed by stimulants, and cocaine (>4%). 4.1% of all males and 1.8% of all females in this age-group meet the DSM-IV criteria for abuse, and 2.5 and 1.6%, respectively, for dependence. Over twice as many overall already have subthreshold diagnoses. With the exception of cannabis, polysubstance use and diagnostic comorbidity are the rule with all types of substance.

Results of 1997 Follow-Up Study of Cannabis Use in 14- to 17-Year-Olds
The following longitudinal analyses focus on the 14- to 17-year-olds from the baseline study [see also ref. 23, 34]. At follow-up a mean 19.6 months after baseline, these subjects were aged 15–19. We confine ourselves to cannabis,

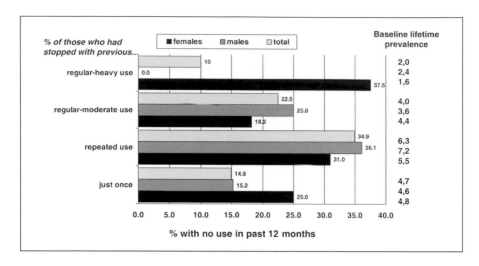

Fig. 7. Transition 1: How many adolescents (14–17 years old) had already stopped the use of cannabis at baseline?

the most commonly used substance, to test the more sophisticated models mentioned at the outset.

Figure 7 (right column) shows the lifetime prevalence of each pattern of use of cannabis found at baseline. The bars in the right column show the percentages of lifetime users reported having remitted in every use pattern class by the time of the baseline study (remitted defined as no further cannabis use in the 12 months before the study). Among regular heavy users, 38% of all females but not a single male subject had ceased use. Corresponding remission rates among regular moderate users were 25% in males, and 18% in females. In those with only light repeated use the remission rates were markedly higher, at 36 and 31%, respectively, and in one-time users we again see very low rates (men 15%, women 25%), perhaps indicating the validity of the rule 'once doesn't count'.

Figure 8 describes the increases in incidence (i.e. new cases in each use pattern category during the follow-up period). In the category of regular heavy users we see an increase especially among men, with an incidence of 2.8%. Increases of 10.3% in men and 7.9% in women are seen for regular moderate use, and 9.2 and 7.6%, respectively, for repeated use, while single first-time use is relatively rare in the now older cohort. These data provide the cumulative lifetime incidences for cannabis use in each of the categories shown in the right numerical table. At follow-up of the originally 14- to 17-year-olds we thus have a cumulative lifetime incidence of 3.8% for regular heavy cannabis

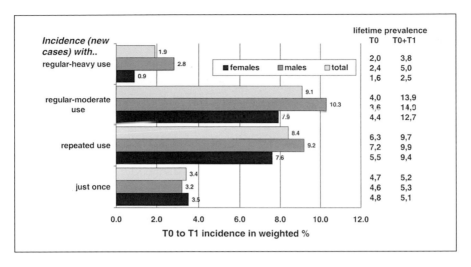

Fig. 8. Transition 2: New cannabis users by patterns of use in the follow-up period: incidence and lifetime prevalence (T0+T1).

Table 3. Transition 3: Changes and stability of cannabis use patterns from T0 to T1: conditional probability

Pattern of use at baseline	Pattern of use at follow-up (T1) in %				
	no	once	repeated	regular-moderate	regular-heavy
No	*82*	4	7	7	1
Just once	47	*5*	19	23	5
Repeated	26	2	*33*	33	6
Regular-moderate	19	0	7	*55*	19
Regular-heavy	15	5	5	55	*20*
Total	74	5	10	14	4

use, 13.9% for regular moderate use, 9.7% for repeated use, and 5.2% for once-only use.

In the follow-up period there was thus a further 10% increase overall in incident cases, so that a total of 32.4% of current 15- to 19-year-olds in Munich have already used cannabis.

Table 3 cross-tabulates use patterns at the baseline and follow-up studies of conditional probabilities. The first row shows that persons who had not

Table 4. Transitions in adolescents: what predicts increasing patterns of use and disorders?

Baseline predictors	Coefficient	z Score	Odds	95% CI
High availability	1.44	6.77***	4.2	2.8–6.4
Diminished will of no use	1.41	7.25**	4.1	2.8–6.0
Lower self-esteem	0.54	2.95**	1.7	1.2–2.5
Alcohol use disorder	0.75	2.33**	2.1	1.1–4.0
Parental substance disorder	0.36	2.19*	1.4	1.0–2.0
Drug use in peer group	0.37	2.04*	1.5	1.0–2.1
Nicotine dependence × age	0.51	2.13**	1.7	1.0–2.7

Cumulative logistic regression (proportional odds model). * = 0.05; ** = 0.01; *** = 0.001.

used cannabis in the baseline study had only a low probability of commencing use by the time of the follow-up study. Those who had used it at least once by the baseline study had already developed a markedly higher probability, especially for regular moderate use at their age level (23%). Repeated users in the initial study remained remarkably stable (33%) with a relatively high risk (again 33%) for regular moderate use. All regular moderate or heavy users are remarkably stable with a tendency to distinctly heavier use patterns and low spontaneous remission rates (19 and 15%, respectively). In other words, this shows us – to our surprise – that in a large proportion of 14- to 17-year-olds, regular cannabis use follows a relatively continuous and stable course, with a tendency to higher use patterns.

Testing Our Model

We have performed empirical statistical tests on the model for our transitional analysis outline at the start of this paper. The model is designed to predict the probability – taking all investigated risk factors into consideration – that persons will show increasing use patterns in the course of their life. The statistical model underpinning this analysis is cumulative logistic regression. It is also known as a proportional odds or risk model and is an innovation among multivariate procedures in that it permits less error-prone hypothesis-based testing of complex association patterns [41–43] (table 4). The result of this complex analysis was highly significant and the model shown to be powerful in that it explains over 62% of the observed variance. Of the large number of risk factors selected by univariate screening, availability proved the most powerful, labile and significant. High availability increases the risk of continuously higher cannabis use and disorder development 4.2-fold. The second factor in the model describes the extent to which a person is certain about not using or ceasing to use cannabis. Interestingly, the distribution of responses showed that almost all those who were absolutely certain that they would either not use cannabis, or would cease using it, did exactly that. Even slight doubt on this point increased the risk of a continuously worse course 4.1-fold. Low self-esteem, combined with few life skills, was the third most important factor, at 1.7. Preexisting alcohol abuse or dependence increased the risk 2.1-fold.

A parental history of substance use disorder, whether smoking, alcohol or drugs, increased the risk of higher and increased patterns of cannabis use in the children. The final two significant predictors in the model were highly correlated with the the first factor (availability), but had additional explanatory value. Friends in the respondents' peer group also was significant in the overall model (OR = 1.5). A significant interaction between age and nicotine dependence (OR = 1.7) indicates that the influence of nicotine dependence seems to increase with age.

Discussion

The data we have collected on the prevalence and incidence of cannabis use indicate that even in regions with high quality of life and low socioeconomic stress indices, such as the greater Munich area, cannabis use is widespread. Contrary to expectations, cannabis use is generally not a one-time or rare event. Rather we find that the probability of transiting to regular prolonged use is clearly higher than that of transiting to cessation.

Particularly striking are the probabilities of transition to polysubstance abuse – above all involving stimulants – even in this young age group of 14- to 17-year-olds. Amphetamine or Ecstasy is usually the second substance used or abused, and even a brief period of repeated or regular use greatly increases the probability of using hallucinogens, especially LSD, in this age group.

Over the average 18-month assessment period between the baseline and follow-up studies, substantially higher risks were also observed for developing abuse and dependence; and while only cannabis abuse and dependence are quantitatively striking, comorbidity with abuse and dependence patterns of other substances must be borne in mind. This mainly involves the development of subthreshold or diagnostically/clinically relevant suprathreshold abuse and dependence syndromes with stimulants, especially Ecstasy, amphetamines and cocaine.

Multivariate longitudinal modeling of these developmental patterns has shown, compared to univariate analyses, that an adequate model can be found which incorporates only relatively few of many significant individual predictors. The strongest predictors are those directly preceding development of the abuse pattern, such as abuse patterns related to legal drugs, especially nicotine and alcohol, and substance availability, whether in a subject's awareness of the supply situation or use of the substances in his peer group. Taken together, these factors constitute a powerful group of predictors for increasing regular and heavy problem use.

Particularly in this age group it is already striking that regular problem substance use is closely related to vulnerabilities based on family genetic predisposition. The simple fact of parental dependence on, or abuse of, a legal substance – interacting with the factors mentioned above – substantially increases the risk of their children proceeding to regular heavy cannabis use. Because of the psychological aspect, there is already a wealth of findings to show that a low level of life skills, poor coping mechanisms and low self-esteem are important determinants for developing problem use of cannabis and probably other substances.

In further analyses we will examine the specific subaspects of this model in detail, and in particular attempt to shed further light on the importance of substance interactions.

References

1   Adlaf EM, Ivis FJ, Smart RG: Ontario Student Drug Use Survey: 1977–1997. Toronto, Addiction Research Foundation, 1997.
2   Anthony JC: Epidemiology of drug dependence and illicit drug use. Curr Opin Psychiary 1991;4: 435–439.
3   Anthony JC, Helzer JE: Epidemiology of drug dependence; in Tsuang MT, Tohen M, Zahner GEP (eds): Textbook in Psychiatric Epidemiology. New York, Wiley, 1995, pp 361–406.
4   Brook JS, Brook DW, Gordon AS, Whiteman M, Cohen P: The psychosocial etiology of adolescent drug use: A family interactional approach. Genet Soc Gen Psychol Monogr 1990;116:111–267.
5   Brook JS, Brook DW, De la Rosa M, Duque LF, Rodriguez E, Montoya ID, Whiteman M: Pathways to marijuana use among adolescents: Cultural/ecological, family, peer, and personal influences. J Am Acad Child Adolesc Psychiatry 1998;37:759–766.
6   Bry BH, McKeon P, Pandina R: Extent of drug use as a function of number of risk factors. J Abnorm Psychol 1982;91:273–279.
7   Clayton RR: Transitions in drug use: Risk and protective factors; in Glantz MD, Pickens R (eds): Vulnerability of Abuse. Washington, American Psychological Association, 1992.
8   Dembo R, Farrow D, Schmeidler J, Burgos W: Testing a causal model of environmental influences on early drug involvement of inner city junior high school youths. Am J Drug Alcohol Abuse 1979; 6:313–336.
9   Edwards RW: Drug and alcohol use among youth in rural communities. NIDA Res Monogr 1997; 168:53–75.
10 Glantz MD: A developmental psychopathology model of drug abuse vulnerability; in Glantz MD, Pickens R (eds): Vulnerability to Drug Abuse. Washington, American Psychological Association, 1992, pp 389–418.

11   Hawkins DJ, Catalano RF, Miller JY: Risk and protective factors for alcohol and other drug problems in adolescence and early adulthood: Implications for substance abuse prevention. Psychol Bull 1992;112:64–105.

12   Kandel DB, Logan JA: Patterns of drug use from adolescence to young adulthood. 1. Periods of risk for initiation, continued use, and discontinuation. AJPH 1984;74:660–672.

13   Kandel DB, Raveis VH: Cessation of illicit drug use in young adulthood. Arch Gen Psychiatry 1989;46:109–116.

14   Kandel DB, Davies M: Progression to regular marijuana involvement: Phenomenology and risk factors for near-daily use; in Glantz D, Pickens R (eds): Vulnerability to Drug Abuse. Washington, American Psychological Association, 1992, pp 211–253.

15   Kandel DB, Faust R: Sequence and stages in patterns of adolescents drug use. Arch Gen Psychiatrie 1975;32:923–932.

16   Kandel DB, Kessler RC, Marguliues RZ: Antecedents and adolescent initiation into stages of drug use: A developmental analysis. J Youth Adolesc 1978;7:13–40.

17   Kaplan HB, Martin SS, Robbins C: Pathways to adolescent drug use: Self-derogation, peer influence, weakening of social controls, and early substance use. J Health Soc Behav 1984;25:270–289.

18   Lettieri DJ: Drug abuse: A review of explanations and models of explanations. Adv Alcohol Subst Abuse 1985;4:9–40.

19   Maddahian E, Newcomb MD, Bentler PM: Adolescent drug use and intention to use drugs: Concurrent and longitudinal analyses of four ethnic groups. Addict Behav 1988;13:191–195.

20   Needle R, Lavee Y, Su S, Brown P, Doherty W: Familial, interpersonal, and interpersonal correlates of drug use: A longitudinal comparison of adolescents in treatment, drug-using adolescents not in treatment, and non-drug-using adolescents. Int J Addict 1988;23:1211–1240.

21   Newcomb MD, Bentler PM: Frequency of sequence of drug use: A longitudinal study from early adolescence to young adulthood. J Drug Educ 1986;16:101–120.

22   Newcomb MD, Maddahian E, Bentler PM: Risk factors for drug use among adolescents: Concurrent and longitudinal analyses. Am J Public Health 1986;76:525–531.

23   Perkonigg A, Lieb R, Höfler M, Sonntag H, Wittchen H-U: Patterns of cannabis use, abuse and dependence in adolescents: Prevalence, incidence and symptom progression. Addiction, in press.

24   Petraitis J, Flay BR, Miller TQ: Reviewing theories of adolescent substance use: Organizing pieces in the puzzle. Psychol Bull 1995;117:67–86.

25   World Health Organization: Tenth Revision of the International Classification of Diseases. ICD-10. Chapter V (F): Menntel and Behavioral Disorders: Diagnostic Criteria for Research. Geneva, World Health Organization, 1991.

26   American Psychiatric Association: Diagnostic and Statistical Manual of Mental Disorders, ed 4. Washington, American Psychiatric Association, 1994.

27   Perkonigg A, Wittchen H-U, Lachner G: Wie häufig sind Substanzmissbrauch und -abhängigkeit? Ein methodenkritischer Überblick. Z Klin Psychol 1996;25:280–295.

28   Lachner G, Wittchen H-U, Perkonigg A, Holly A, Schuster P, Wunderlich U, Türk D, Garczynski E, Pfister H: Structure, content and reliability of the Munich-Composite International Diagnostic Interview (M-CIDI). Substance use sections. Eur Addict Res 1998;4:28–41.

29   Perkonigg A, Lieb R, Wittchen H-U: Substance use, abuse and dependence in Germany: A review of selected epidemiological data. Eur Addict Res 1998;4:8–17.

30   Perkonigg A, Lieb R, Wittchen H-U: Prevalence of use, abuse and dependence of illicit drugs among adolescents and young adults in a community sample. Eur Addict Res 1998;4:58–66.

31   Wittchen H-U, Nelson CB: Early developmental stages of substance abuse. Eur Addict Res 1998;4:83.

32   Wittchen H-U, Perkonigg A, Lachner G, Nelson CB: Early developmental stages of psychopathology study (EDSP): Objectives and design. Eur Addict Res 1998;4:18–27.

33   Holly A, Türk D, Nelson CB, Pfister H, Wittchen H-U: Prävalenz von Alkoholkonsum, Alkoholmissbrauch und -abhängigkeit bei Jugendichen und jungen Erwachsenen. Z Klin Psychol 1997;66:171–178.

34   Wittchen H-U, Höfler M, Perkonigg A, Sonntag H, Lieb R: Wie stabil sind Drogenkonsum und das Auftreten klinisch-diagnostisch relevanter Missbrauchs- und Abhängigkeitsstadien bei Jugendlichen? Eine epidemiologische Studie am Beispiel von Cannabis. Kindheit Entwicklung 1998;7:188–198.

35 Wittchen H-U, Nelson GB, Lachner G: Prevalence of mental disorders and psychosocial impairments in adolescents and young adults. Psychol Med 1998;28:109–126.

36 Wittchen H-U, Pfister H (eds): DIA-X-Interviews: Manual für Screening-Verfahren und Interview; Interviewheft Längsschnittuntersuchung (DIA-X-Lifetime); Ergänzungsheft (DIA-X-Lifetime); Interviewheft Querschnittuntersuchung (DIA-X-12 Monate); Ergänzungsheft (DIA-X-12Monate); PC-Programm zur Durchführung des Interviews (Längs- und Querschnittuntersuchung); Auswertungsprogramm. Frankfurt, Swets & Zeitlinger, 1997.

37 Lachner G, Wittchen H-U: Münchener Composite International Diagnostic Interview, M-CIDI (familiengenetische Version), Elternabefragung, Version 2.0. München: Max-Planck-Institut für Psychiatrie, 1997.

38 Lieb R, Lachner G, Sonntag H, Pfister H, Höfler M, Gander F, Wittchen H-U: Zwischenbericht zum Projektteil «Familiengenetik und familiäre Sozialisation» im Rahmen des Forschungsvorhabens «Vulnerabilitäts- und Protektionsfaktoren bei Frühstadien von Substanzmissbrauch und -abhängigkeit: Eine Verlaufsstudie», gefördert vom BMFBW, Laufzeit. 1.7.1994 bis 31.3.1999. Förderkennzeichen 01 EB9405, Berichtzeitraum: 1.8.1996 bis 30.4.1998. München, Max-Planck-Institut für Psychiatrie, 1998.

39 McCullagh P: Regression model for ordinal data (with discussion). J R Stat Soc 1980;B42:109–127.

40 Perkonigg A, Beloch E, Garczynski E, Nelson CB, Pfister H, Wittchen H-U: Prävalenz von Drogenmissbrauch und -abhängigkeit bei Jugendlichen und jungen Erwachsenen: Gebrauch, Diagnosen und Auftreten erster Missbrauchs- und Abhängigkeitsmerkmale. Z Klin Psychol 1997;26:247–257.

41 Fahrmeir A, Tutz G: Multivariate Statistical Modelling Based on Generalized Linear Models. Berlin, Springer, 1994.

42 Höfler M, Lieb R, Perkonigg A, Schuster P, Sonntag H, Wittchen H-U: Covariates of cannabis use progression patterns in a representative population sample of adolescents: A prospective examination of vulnerability and risk factors. Addiction, in press.

43 Liang K-Y, Zeger S: Longitudinal data analyses using Generalized Linear Models. Biometrica 1986; 73:13–22.

Prof. Dr. Hans-Ulrich Wittchen, Max-Planck-Institut für Psychiatrie,
Kraepelinstrasse 10, D–80804 München (Germany)
Tel. +49 89 30622-546, Fax +49 89 30622-544, E-Mail wittchen@mpipsykl.mpg.de

Ladewig D (ed): Basic and Clinical Science of Substance Related Disorders.
Bibl Psychiatr. Basel, Karger, 1999, No 168, pp 23–28

....

Aspects of the Psychosocial Consequences and Biological Evaluation of Heroin Treatments

R. Stohler

Psychiatrische Universitätsklinik, Sektor West, Zürich, Switzerland

This paper presents some of the relevant findings generated mainly in Basel in collaboration with the patients of the Janus Project. The Janus Project is the Basel treatment center where medically prescribed intravenous heroin, morphine and methadone are dispensed to severely addicted opiate users in the context of the Swiss national PROVE study [1].

We now have the Summary Report by Uchtenhagen [2] on the PROVE projects, together with the supplementary data combined in the *Final Report on the Effects of Narcotic Prescription on Delinquency in Drug Addicts* by Killias and Rabasa [3]. Anyone requiring a more detailed exposition of the topic is referred to these reports.

In various studies in Basel we examined the 'biological' effect of heroin and also the psychological consequences of these treatments. The teams and their members were: the Dependence Disorder Group of Basel University of Psychiatry of D. Ladewig, K. Dürsteler, I. Hug, P. Hruz, E. Mark, J. Sattler-Mayr, F. Schellenberg and R. Stohler; the Psychogeriatrics Group of F. Müller-Spahn, R. Störmer, M. von Arx and C. Hock; the Somatic Medicine Group of R. Ritz, M. Battegay, P. Haller, A. Scholer and W. Strobel, and the Neurology Group of R. Kocher, R. Mager, J. Loosli and M. Schmidlin.

Pharmacokinetics of Heroin

The first step studying the biological effects of heroin was to determine the pharmacokinetics of the drug and its metabolites. In the Intensive Care Unit of Basel University Hospital, 15 patients injected themselves with medically prescribed heroin. Plasma levels of heroin and it metabolites (among other parameters not discussed here) were determined 5 min before and 5, 15, 30, 60, 120, 240 and 360 min after injection. The data have not yet been fully evaluated. At present, though, I can say that the plasma half-life of diacetylmorphine could be determined in only 2 subjects, and was 3.5 min in both cases. In the other subjects the half life was so short that heroin was no longer detectable at the second data point, so that the kinetics could not be calculated. 6-Monoacetylmorphine was readily assayable in 11 subjects and had a plasma half-life of 9 ± 3.5 min, with a range of 3.4–17.5 min. Calculations still need to be done to determine the extent to which rush, euphoria, withdrawal symptoms and attention correlate with the plasma concentration-time curves of individual metabolites.

Electroencephalography

Just a few months after the start of the project in Basel, we became concerned about the occurrence of epileptic seizures in the participants. We therefore recorded EEGs and ECGs before, during and up to about 45 min after heroin, morphine and methadone injection. Proconvulsive activity has been described for opioids in the literature. Various authors postulate mediation of (naloxone-sensitive) epileptic activity by μ- or δ-opiate receptors [4]. However, a (non-naloxone-sensitive) interaction of high-dose systemically administered morphine at the GABA receptor has also been discussed as an alternative or additional mechanism [5]. Our team also considered postinjection cerebral hypoxia as a possible cause. Nineteen subjects from the Basel Janus Project (including 5 patients with epileptic seizures during treatment in the project) participated in the study. 'The results of the study were mixed, encompassing normal EEG recordings in 6 patients before and after injection, mildly pathological preinjection EEG with no change postinjection in 5 patients, and marked signs of hypersynchronous activity or even pathognomonic epileptiform discharges postinjection in 8 patients (including 2 epileptics). These abnormalities were not observed in the methadone group' [6].

Etiological Research

In an as yet unpublished pilot study, we looked further into the causes of the frequently present neuronal hyperexcitability. In collaboration with the Psychogeriatrics Group, we used near-infrared spectroscopy (NIRS) to measure cortical oxy- and deoxyhemaglobin in 10 subjects before and after

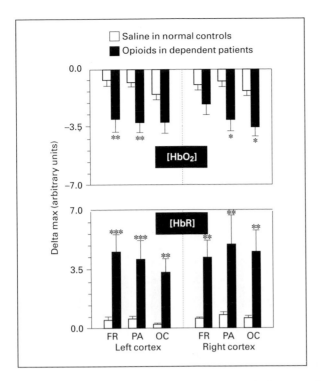

Fig. 1. Effects of i.v. opioids (heroin, methadone) on [HbO$_2$] and [HbR] in opioid-dependent subjects compared to the effects of i.v. saline in control subjects. Pairwise comparisons of each single region were done with U tests (FR = frontal, PA = parietal, OC = occipital). Values are means $\pm$ SEM of Δmax throughout a period of 420 s after injection (* p < 0.05, ** p < 0.01. *** p < 0.001).

heroin injection and in 2 patients taking intravenous methadone. Ten age-matched non-opiate-dependent staff members served as controls.

We observed an unexpectedly large rise in deoxyhemoglobin and a fall in oxyhemoglobin. Figure 1 shows the maximum increases and falls in hemoglobin relative to 10 controls injected with normal saline. Heroin and methadone patients did not differ in this investigation. Possible explanations included increased oxygen extraction by hyperactive cortical neurons, but also decreased oxyhemoglobin delivery. Using pulse oximetry, we therefore monitored oxygen saturation for 3 h in 9 patients maintained on relatively high i.v. methadone doses. There was a maximum fall to 95% (fig. 2). However, a different picture emerged in a patient maintained on 300 mg of heroin whose oxygen saturation fell to worrying levels during simultaneous NIRS and pulse oximetry (fig. 3). It thus remains to be investigated what happens immediately after heroin

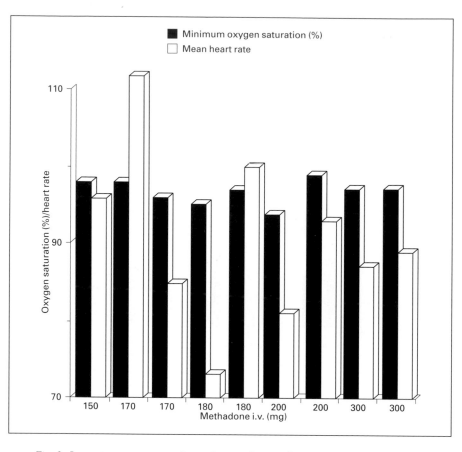

Fig. 2. Lowest oxygen saturation values and mean heart rate in 9 patients of an i.v. methadone maintenance treatment program. After having received the prescribed methadone dose patients were monitored by pulsoxymetry for 1 h.

injection. An interesting question is also the rush or flash phenomenon, on which there are no studies to be found in the scientific literature. Figure 3 shows simultaneous recordings of [HbO$_2$] and [HbR] by NIRS (fig. 3a) and pulse oximetry (fig. 3b) in a 'typical' patient maintained on 300 mg of heroin twice daily. Figure 3c shows the typical pattern of a control on saline infusion.

Psychosocial Consequences

Nevertheless we were able to reduce the number of seizures during the course of the project by treating the patients for example with anticonvulsants,

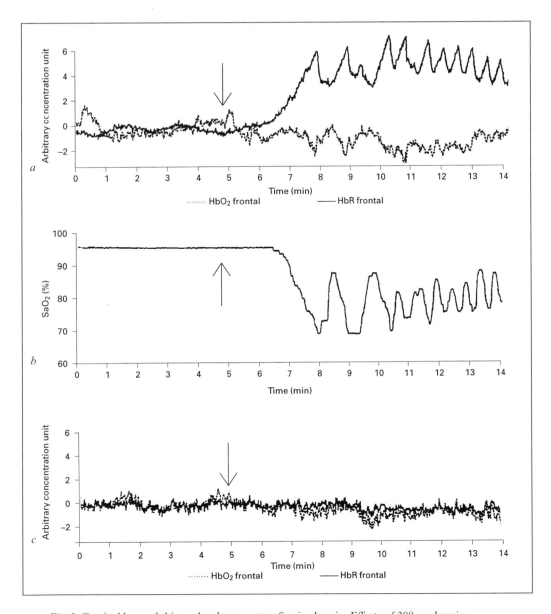

Fig. 3. Cortical hemoglobin and pulsoxymetry after i.v. heroin. Effects of 300 mg heroin on [HbO₂] and [HbR] in the frontal cortex (*a*) and on simultaneously registered oxygen saturation (*b*) of a representative opioid-dependent subject. In comparison, *c* shows the effects of intravenous saline on [HbO₂] and [HbR] in the frontal cortex of a representative control subject. Arrows indicate time of injection.

treatments that only became possible in the context of these projects [8]. Because of their participation in the Janus Project, patients had increased access to somatic treatment at Basel University Hospital. As Ms. Haller showed in her paper on treatment costs in 34 Janus patients comparing 2 years before and 1 year after starting in the project, admissions to the emergency ward of Basel University Hospital – mostly referrals from the project – increased from 1.6 to 2.2 (year before project entry vs. 1st year in project). By contrast, inpatient treatments declined from 1.5 to 1 and length of hospital stay from 16.4 to 10.7 days, reducing hospital costs from SFr. 21,708 to 13,567 [9].

References

1   Schweizerischer Bundesrat; Verordnung über die Förderung der wissenschaftlichen Begleitforschung zur Drogenprävention und Verbesserung der Lebensbedingungen Drogenabhängiger. Schweizerischer Bundesrat, 1992.
2   Uchtenhagen A: Synthesebericht. Zürich, Institut fur Suchtforschung/Institut für Sozial- und Präventivmedizin der Universität, 1997.
3   Killias M, Rabasa J: Schlussbericht zu den Auswirkungen der Verschreibung von Betäubungsmitteln auf die Delinquenz von Drogenabhängigen. Lausanne, Institut de police scientifique et de criminologie, 1997.
4   Reisine T, Pasternak G: Opioid analgesics and antagonists; in Hardman JG, Gilman AG, Limbird LE (eds): Goodman and Gilman's the Pharmacological Basis of Therapeutics, ed 9. New York, Pergamon, 1996.
5   Sagratella S, Scotti-de Carolis A: In vivo and in vitro epileptogenic effects of the enkephalinergic system. Ann 1st Super Sanità 1993;29:413–418.
6   Hug I: Epileptiforme Störungen bei opiatabhängigen Patienten under intravenöser Substitutionstherapie mit Heroin, Morphin und Methadon; Diss Universität Basel, 1997, p 117.
7   Hock C, Villringer K, Müller-Spahn F, Wenzel R, Heekeren H, Schuh-Hofer S, Hofmann M, Minoshima S, Schwaiger M, Dirnagl U, Villringer A: Decrease in parietal cerebral hemoglobin oxygenation during performance of a verbal fluency task in patients with Alzheimer's disease monitored by means of near-infrared spectroscopy (NIRS): Correlation with simultaneous rCBF PET measurements. Brain Res 1997;755:293–303.
8   Uchtenhagen A, Gutzwiller F, Dobler-Mikola A, Steffen T: Programme for a medical prescription of narcotics: A synthesis of results. Eur Addict Res 1997;3:160–163.
9   Haller P: Verbesserung der medizinischen Versorgung Opiatabhängiger durch die ärztlich kontrollierte Abgabe von Heroin; med Diss Basel, 1996.

Dr. Rudolf Stohler, Psychiatrische Universitätsklinik, Sektor West,
Militärstrasse 8, Postfach 1930, CH–8021 Zürich (Switzerland)
Tel. +41 1 291 12 40, Fax +41 1 291 12 40, E-Mail stohler@spd.unizh.ch

Ladewig D (ed): Basic and Clinical Science of Substance Related Disorders.
Bibl Psychiatr. Basel, Karger, 1999, No 168, pp 29–39

....

Comorbidity Research in Substance Use Disorders

Martin Preisig[a], *Brenda T. Fenton*[b]

[a] University Psychiatric Hospital, Lausanne, Switzerland;
[b] University Psychiatric Hospital, Geneva, Switzerland

The use of illicit substances and excessive alcohol are major public health issues which have gained increasing interest in research during the last two decades. One important finding of this research has been the high comorbidity of alcoholism and drug disorders with a wide range of other psychiatric conditions. This paper provides (1) epidemiological data on the magnitude of the comorbidity between substance use disorders and other psychiatric conditions and (2) results of research in genetic epidemiology aimed at determining the nature of the association underlying this comorbidity.

Despite the difficulties inherent in the assessment of the prevalence of substance disorders due to issues of social desirability and confidentiality, recent surveys conducted in several Western countries revealed high lifetime prevalence of alcohol abuse/dependence: 14.1% of the US population met DSM-III-R criteria for alcohol dependence [Kessler et al., 1994] and 13.0% of the West German population were found to meet criteria for alcohol abuse or dependence [Wittchen et al., 1992]. Although population-based estimates for substance use disorders are not available in Switzerland, 7% of the population experienced problems with others due to their drinking or received requests from others to reduce their drinking [Fahrenkrug and Müller, 1989; ISPA, 1993]. Approximately 5% of all deaths and 10% of all car accidents in Switzerland are attributable to alcohol [ISPA, 1993].

Based on available international data through 1990, Switzerland had one of the highest drug-related death rates with 6 deaths per 100,000 persons [Fahrenkrug et al., 1995]. In 1991 and 1992 drugs were the second largest cause of mortality for persons aged 15–24, with the largest proportion of deaths in the 20–30 age range [Schick and Alberto, 1994]. The mortality rate of opiate-dependent persons has been estimated at 20–30 per 1,000, which is 10–30 times that of the general population [Buschor and Wessel, 1983]. The introduction of AIDS resulted in a steep increase in the number of deaths of drug addicts from the late 1980s to present [Parma Information, 1996]. The risk of AIDS among drug users, specifically intravenous drug users, increases the negative impact of drug use on both individuals and society. Indeed, in 1993 an estimated 33% of male and 60% of female AIDS cases in Switzerland were intravenous drug users.

In the late 1980s, Switzerland had a higher than average European prevalence of both cannabis and hard drug consumption [Reuband, 1995]. In the past decade, estimates of illicit drug use have ranged from 21 to 29% for persons aged 17–30, whereas the rate for older persons (aged 31–45) was 10–14%. The prevalence of opioid users in the age group 15–25 was estimated at 3% from 1971 to 1990 [Binder et al., 1979; Müller, 1982; IUMSP Lausanne/IPSO Zurich, 1990] and 1.3% within an extended age range (ages 15–39) for the period 1990–1993 [Rehm, 1995]. With respect to regular hard drug use (either heroin or cocaine), the number of addicts was estimated to be between 30,000 and 50,000 persons in the mid 1990s, up from 25,000 persons in 1989 [ISPA, 1993; Fahrenkrug et al., 1995; Estermann, 1996].

Comorbidity of Substance Use Disorders and Other Psychiatric Conditions

Comorbidity between Alcohol and Drug Disorders

The most frequent pattern of drug abuse is polysubstance abuse [Rounsaville 1988]. High lifetime comorbidity of alcohol and drug disorders has been observed in both clinical [Khantzian and Treece, 1985; Rounsaville et al., 1991] and epidemiological studies [Regier et al., 1990]. In both types of studies, a higher degree of comorbidity with alcoholism has been observed in cocaine addicts as compared to their opioid-addicted counterparts [Regier et al., 1990; Rounsaville et al., 1991].

Comorbidity of Substance and Other Psychiatric Disorders

A summary of the rates of comorbidity of selected disorders with alcohol and drug dependence from major epidemiological samples is presented in table 1. The association between alcoholism and mood disorders observed in many clinical studies has been confirmed by studies of community [Weissman and Myers, 1980; Boyd et al., 1984; Helzer and Pryzbeck, 1988; Regier et al.,

Table 1. Psychiatric comorbidity with alcohol and drug dependence in community samples

Disorder	Alcohol dependence			Drug dependence		
	ECA[a]	NCS[b]	Zurich[c]	ECA[a]	NCS[b]	Zurich[c]
MDD	2.3	2.7	2.0	3.7	2.8	2.6
Bipolar	4.6	9.7	2.3[d]	8.3	8.4	4.6[d]
ASPD	14.7	11.7	–	15.6	14.2	–
Panic	3.3	2.0	1.4	4.4	3.8	1.4
GAD	–	2.8	0.4	–	3.8	0.6
Social phobia	all	2.2	3.5	all	2.6	2.1
Agoraphobia	phobia	1.7	0.6	phobia	2.8	1.9
Simple phobia	*1.6*	2.1	1.4	*2.2*	2.5	1.4

ASPD = Antisocial Personality Disorder; GAD = Generalized Anxiety Disorder; MDD = Major Depressive Disorder.

[a] Regier et al. [1990].
[b] Kessler et al. [1996].
[c] Angst [1993].
[d] Hypomania.

1990; Angst, 1993; Kendler et al., 1993; Kessler et al., 1996]. Bipolar disorder (range of odds ratios: 2.3–14.5) has been found to be more strongly associated with alcoholism than major depressive disorder (range of odds ratios: 1.3–4.1). An association between alcohol disorders and anxiety disorders has also been observed in both clinical [Lader, 1972; Woodruff et al., 1972; Marks and Lader, 1973; Mullaney and Trippett, 1979; Bowen et al., 1984; Smail ct al., 1984; Weiss and Rosenberg, 1985; Bibb and Chambless, 1986; Ross et al., 1988; Kushner et al., 1990; Regier et al., 1990; Angst, 1993; Kessler et al., 1996]. In general, comorbidity in clinical patients with anxiety disorders and alcoholism is substantially greater for alcohol dependence than for abuse [Mullaney and Trippett, 1979; Bowen et al., 1984; Smail et al., 1984; Stockwell et al., 1984; Hesselbrock et al., 1985; Roelofs, 1985; Weiss et al., 1986; Ross et al., 1988].

A high comorbidity with mood disorders has also been observed in clinical samples of opioid addicts [Khantzian and Treece, 1985; Rounsaville et al., 1991] and cocaine abusers [Gawin and Kleber, 1986; Weiss et al., 1986]. Cocaine/stimulant disorders were found to be associated with both types of mood disorders, whereas opioid disorders only with major [Khantzian and Treece, 1985; Dackis et al., 1986; Rounsaville et al., 1991]. The high comorbidity between drug and mood disorders was also found in epidemiological studies

[Regier et al., 1990; Angst, 1993; Kessler et al., 1996]. Again, bipolar disorder has been shown to have a higher comorbidity with dependence on any psychoactive drug than major depression [Regier et al., 1990; Angst, 1993; Brady and Sonne, 1995; Kessler et al., 1996; Wiffchen et al., 1996]. Most of the clinical and epidemiological studies also found associations between drug and specific anxiety disorders [Quitkin et al., 1972; Mirin et al., 1988, 1991].

Underlying Mechanisms of the Association between Substance Use Disorders and Other Pychiatric Conditions

The nature of the association between substance and other psychiatric disorders remains to be elucidated. The exploration of the mechanisms of comorbidity requires an interdisciplinary approach and study designs beyond the scope of clinical and cross-sectional epidemiological studies, which so far have comprised the bulk of comorbidity research. Powerful tools to determine the mechanisms of association are family, adoption and twin studies, since these study designs can provide clues as to whether an association is causal or due to shared underlying etiology. Such studies can be combined with genetic association studies to identify the molecular basis of the association.

Within the family study paradigm, if a true association exists between two disorders, there are two general mechanisms by which it may occur: (1) either one of the disorders could cause or predispose to the other, or (2) both conditions could share underlying etiologic factors [Merikangas and Gelernter, 1990. If one disorder causes the other, we would expect that the relatives of a diseased person would manifest an increased risk of the causal disorder and the combination of the two syndromes, but not the pure form of the other disorder. For example, if mood disorders cause alcoholism, relatives of probands with mood disorders should have an increased rate of alcoholism, but only in the presence of a lifetime history of mood disorder. In contrast, if two disorders are manifestations of the same underlying factors, relatives of probands with pure forms of either disorder should have elevated rates of pure forms of the other disorder as compared to population rates. Therefore, relatives of probands suffering from mood disorder alone should have an increased risk of pure alcoholism and the converse.

The Nature of the Association between Alcohol and Drug Disorders

A central question in the substance abuse field has been whether there is a general risk for addiction which underlies both alcohol and drug disorders or whether different pathways of risk exist for each type of substance disorder. The existing family and adoption studies provide contradictory evidence regarding the nature of the association between alcohol and drug disorders. The majority of family studies suggest independent transmission of alcohol and drug disorders [Hill et al., 1977; Rounsaville et al., 1982; Mirin et al., 1984; Gfroerer, 1987; Meller et al., 1988; Mirin et al., 1988; Stabenau, 1992; Preisig and Merikangas 1996]. However, one family study [Schuckit, 1985] and an adoption study [Cadoret et al., 1995] provide some evidence for common etiologic factors for the two types of substance disorders.

The Nature of the Association between Alcoholism and Other Psychiatric Disorders

Alcohol and Mood Disorder

There are many family history studies, family studies and offspring studies of probands suffering from affective disorders or alcoholism. However, the question of whether or not affective disorders and alcoholism share etiologic factors has yet to be resolved. Limitations of most studies include the absence of an appropriate control group or the lack of distinction between 'pure' and combined forms of the two conditions among either probands or their relatives.

Two early family studies of alcoholics with normal controls [Amark, 1951; Bleuler, 1995] which showed an increased risk of affective disorders among relatives of alcoholic probands suggest a common etiology for these two conditions. In contrast to this finding, a more recent controlled family study [Maier and Merikangas, 1996] as well as three studies comparing the risk of depression in the relatives of alcoholics with that of relatives of primary depressives [Winokur et al., 1971; Cloninger et al., 1979; Schuckit, 1985] suggest the independent transmission of the two syndromes. Similarly, studies comparing the families of probands with unipolar depression to those of normal controls [Gershon et al., 1975, 1982; Merikangas et al., 1985, 1994; Maier and Merikangas, 1996] as well as studies comparing the families of probands suffering from primary unipolar depression to those of primary alcoholics [Lewis et al., 1986; Grove et al., 1987] generally do not provide evidence for shared liability between the two conditions. This has also been confirmed in a recent family study [Nelson et al., 1995] which, however, did not conduct separate transmission analyses for relatives of unipolar and bipolar probands. Only one controlled family study with major depressive probands [Winokur and Coryell, 1991] provides some support for shared etiologic factors between unipolar depression and alcohol disorders with higher rates of alcoholism among the relatives of female depressives as compared to the relatives of female controls.

Among the few controlled family studies on bipolar disorders, three suggest independent transmission of alcoholism and bipolar disorder [Gershon et al., 1975; Dunner et al., 1979; Gershon et al., 1982] and two provided some evidence for shared etiologic factors between bipolar and alcohol disorder [Cassidy et al., 1957; Maier and Merikangas, 1996]. Cassidy et al. [1957] reported a higher risk of alcoholism for male relatives of bipolars as compared to male relatives of controls. The results of a recent family study [Maier and Merikangas, 1996] obtained by two different statistical methods were not in full agreement regarding the relationship between bipolar disorder and alcoholism. The proportional hazards models found no significant impact of one of the two disorders in the proband on the risk for the alternate disorder in the relatives, whereas the results of the bivariate polygenic threshold model of cosegregation suggested a modest covariation between familial components underlying both disorders. In the study of Winokur et al. [1993] relatives of 'pure' bipolar probands were found at a higher risk for alcohol disorders than those of 'pure' unipolar depressives controlling for the presence of comorbid affective disorders in relatives. This would suggest that shared etiologic factors are more likely to exist between alcohol and bipolar disorder than between alcohol and major depressive disorders.

Alcohol and Anxiety Disorders

Although the familial aggregation of both alcohol [Cotton, 1979; Begleiter and Porjesz, 1988; Devor and Cloninger, 1989] and anxiety disorders [Cohen et al., 1951; Noyes et al., 1978; Crowe et al., 1983] has been demonstrated in numerous studies, only a few have systematically and simultaneously examined the patterns of cosegregation of both these disorders among first-degree relatives of affected probands. Numerous family studies of both alcoholism [Merikangas et al., 1985] and anxiety disorders [Cohen et al., 1951; Noyes et al., 1978; Munjack and Moss, 1981; Harris et al., 1983; Leckman et al., 1983] have reported elevated rates of the other condition among relatives. However, because these studies did not stratify probands and relatives according to comorbid disorders, they cannot provide information about the nature of the association between anxiety and alcoholism. In the recent findings of Merikangas et al. [1998], panic disorder in probands predicted alcoholism in relatives but not the converse, thereby supporting a model of partially shared liability. In contrast, the association between alcoholism and social phobia appeared to be causal in nature.

Drug and Mood Disorders

The results of the few available family studies on the association between mood disorders and substance abuse other than alcohol are contradictory. Preliminary studies of drug abusers suggested shared etiology for drug and bipolar disorder [Mirin et al., 1984; Gershon et al., 1988], whereas a family history study [Rounsaville et al., 1991] on treated cocaine and opioid addicts found no such evidence. With respect to unipolar depression, first-degree relatives of treated opioid and cocaine addicts had an increased risk of major depression, after adjusting for comorbidity in the proband [Rounsaville et al., 1991]. Two family studies of mood probands provide evidence for independent transmission of mood and drug disorders [Gershon et al., 1982; Schuckit, 1985].

Drug and Anxiety Disorders

The few available family studies of substance abusers have demonstrated specificity of transmission of drug and anxiety disorders [Rounsaville et al., 1991; Fenton and Merikangas, 1996].

Conclusions

Clinical and epidemiological studies reveal substance use disorders to be highly associated with each other and with a wide range of other psychiatric conditions. Family, adoption and twin studies are powerful tools to elucidate the mechanisms of the association, since these study designs can provide clues as to whether an association is causal or due to shared underlying etiology.

Existing methodologically rigorous studies generally provide evidence for the independent transmission of specific alcohol and drug disorders. They also generally support independent transmission of alcoholism and major depression. However, shared etiology cannot be ruled out in the association of alcoholism and bipolar disorder. The nature of the association between alcoholism and anxiety appears to depend upon the specific anxiety disorder. The comorbidity of panic disorder and alcohol dependence may be due to shared etiologic factors, whereas that of social phobia and alcohol dependence is likely to be causal. The few rigorous studies on the association of drug, mood and anxiety disorders do not yet provide sufficiently consistent results to draw definitive conclusions about the nature of the associations between these disorders. The results of the existing studies need further confirmation, particularly with respect to drug disorders. Future family studies should be combined with molecular genetic approaches, such as association and linkage studies, to identify the molecular genetic basis of the postulated mechanism of the association.

References

Amark C: A study in alcoholism. Acta Psychiatr Scand 1951;70(suppl):283.
Angst J: Comorbidity of anxiety, phobia, compulsion and depression. Int Clin Psychopharmacol 1993; 8(suppl 1):21–25.
Begleiter H, Porjesz B: Potential biological markers in individuals at high risk for alcoholism. Alcohol Clin Exp Res 1988;12:488–493.
Bibb JL, Chambless DL: Alcohol use and abuse among diagnosed agoraphobics. Behav Res Ther 1986; 24:49–58.
Binder J, Sieber M, Angst J: Development of narcotics consumption in adolescents 19 and 20 years old: A comparison in the canton of Zurich 1971, 1979 and 1978. Schweiz Med Wochenschr 1979;109: 1298–1305.
Bleuler M: Familial and personal background in chronic alcoholics; in Diethelm O (ed): Etiology of Chronic Alcoholism. Springfield, Thomas, 1955, pp 110–166.
Bohman M, Sigvardsson S, Cloninger DR: Maternal inheritance of alcohol abuse: Cross-fostering analysis of adopted women. Arch Gen Psychiatry 1981;38:965–969.
Bowen RC, Cipywnyk D, D'Arcy C, Keegan D: Alcoholism, anxiety disorders and agoraphobia. Alcohol Clin Exp Res 1984;8:48–51.
Boyd JH, Burke JD, Gruenberg E, Holzer CE 3d, Rae DS, George LK, Karno M, Stoltzman R, McEvoy L, Nestadt G: Exclusion criteria of DSM-III: A study of co-occurrence of hierarchy-free syndromes. Arch Gen Psychiatry 1984;41:983–989.
Brady KT, Sonne SC: The relationship between substance abuse and bipolar disorder. J Clin Psychiatry 1995;56:19–24.
Buschor F, Wessel J: Überlebensquote Drogenabhängiger: Langzeitanalyse bei 530 Ambulanzklienten der Zugangsjahre 1969 bis 1977. Dtsch Med Wochenschr 1983;108:1345–1351.
Cadoret RJ, Yates WR, Troughton E, Woolworth G, Stewart MA: Adoption study demonstrating two genetic pathways to drug abuse. Arch Gen Psychiatry 1995;52:42–52.
Cassidy WL, Flanagan NB, Spellman M, Cohen ME: Clinical observations in manic depressive disease. JAMA 1957;164:1535–1546.
Cloninger CR, Reich T, Wetzel R: Alcoholism and affective disorders: Familial association and genetic models; in Goodwin DW, Erickson CK (eds): Alcoholism and Affective Disorders: Clinical, Genetic and Biochemical Studies. New York, SP Medical and Scientific Books, 1957, pp 57–86.
Cohen ME, Badal DW, Kilpatrick A, Reed EW, White PD: The high familial prevalence of neuro-circulatory asthenia (anxiety neurosis, effort syndrome). Am J Hum Genet 1951;3:126–158.
Cotton NS: The familial incidence of alcoholism: A review. J Stud Alcohol 1979;40:89–116.
Crowe RR, Noyes R, Pauls DL, Slymen D: A family study of panic disorder. Arch Gen Psychiatry 1983; 40:1065–1069.
Dackis CA, Gold MS, Pottash AL, Sweeney DR: Evaluating depression in alcoholics. Psychiatry Res 1986;17:105–109.
Devor EJ, Cloninger CR: Genetics of alcoholism. Annu Rev Genet 1989;23:19–36.
Dunner DL, Hensel BM, Fieve RR: Bipolar illness: Factors in drinking behavior. Am J Psychiatry 1979; 136:583–585.
Estermann J: Sozialepidemiologie des Drogenkonsums: Zu Prävalenz und Inzidenz des Heroin- und Kokaingebrauchs und dessen polizeiliche Verfolgung. Berlin, Verlag für Wissenschaft und Bildung, 1996.
Fahrenkrug H, Müller R: Alkohol und Gesundheit in der Schweiz. Lausanne, ISPA/SFA, 1989.

Fahrenkrug H, Rehm, Müller R, Klingemann H, Linder R: Drogues illégales en Suisse 1990–1993: La situation dans les cantons et en Suisse. Institut suisse de prévention de l'alcoolisme et autres toxicomanies (ISPA). Zürich, Seismo, 1995.

Fenton BT, Merikangas KR: Comorbidity and co-transmission of substance and anxiety disorders; in Symp Comorbidity in Families: Mechanisms and Treatment. Am Psychiatr Assoc Meet, New York City, May 1996.

Gawin FH, Kleber HD: Abstinence symptomatology and psychiatric diagnosis in cocaine abusers: Clinical observations. Arch Gen Psychiatry 1986;43:190–213.

Gershon ES, Mark A, Cohen N, Belizon N, Baron M, Knobe K: Transmitted factors in the morbid risk of affective disorders: A controlled study. J Psychiat Res 1975;12:283–299.

Gershon ES, Hamovit J, Guroff JJ, Dibble E, Leckman JF, Sceery W, Targum SD, Nurnberger JI Jr, Goldin LR, Bunney WE Jr: A family study of schizoaffective, bipolar I, bipolar II, unipolar and normal probands. Arch Gen Psychiatry 1982;39:1157–1167.

Gershon ES, DeLisi LE, Hamovit J, Nurnberger JI Jr, Maxwell ME, Schreiber J, Dauphinais D, Dingman CW, Guroff JJ: A controlled family study of chronic psychoses: Schizophrenia and schizoaffective disorder. Arch Gen Psychiatry 1988;45:328–336.

Gfroerer J: Correlation between drug use by teenagers and drug use by older family members. Am J Drug Alcohol Abuse 1987;13:95–108.

Grove WM, Andreasen NC, Winokur G, Clayton PJ, Endicott J, Coryell WH: Primary and secondary affective disorders: Unipolar patients compared on familial aggregation. Compr Psychiatry 1987;28:113–126.

Harris EL, Noyes R Jr, Crowe RR, Chaudhry DR: Family study of agoraphobia: Report of a pilot study. Arch Gen Psychiatry 1983;40:1061–1064.

Helzer JE, Pryzbeck TR: The co-occurrence of alcoholism with other psychiatric disorders in the general population and its impact on treatment. J Stud Alcohol 1988;49:219–224.

Hesselbrock MN, Meyer RE, Keener JJ: Psychopathology in hospitalized alcoholics. Arch Gen Psychiatry 1985;42:1050–1055.

Hill SY, Cloninger RC, Ayre FR: Independent familial transmission of alcoholism and opiate abuse. Alcohol Clin Exp Res 1977;1:335–342.

Institut suisse de prevention de l'alcoolisme et autres toxicomanies: Chiffres et Données sur L'Alcool et les Autres Drogues. Lausanne, ISPA, 1993.

Institut universitaire de médecine sociale et préventive, Lausanne IPSO, Zürich, 1990.

Kendler KS, Heath AC, Neale MC, Kessler RC, Eaves LJ: Alcoholism and major depression in women: A twin study of the causes of comorbidity. Arch Gen Psychiatry 1993;50:590–698.

Kessler RC, McGonagle KA, Zhao S, Nelson CB, Hughes M, Eshleman S, Wittchen HU, Kendler K: Lifetime and 12 month prevalence of DSM-III-R psychiatric disorders in the United States. Arch Gen Psychiatry 1994;51:8–19.

Keesler RC, Nelson CB, McGonagle KA, Edlund MJ, Frank RG, Leaf PJ: The epidemiology of co-occurring addictive and mental disorders in the National Comorbidity Survey: Implications for prevention and service utilization. Am I Orthopsychiatry 1996;66:17–31.

Khantzian EJ, Treece C: DSM-III psychiatric diagnosis of narcotic addicts. Arch Gen Psychiatry 1985;42:1067–1071.

Kushner MG, Sher KJ, Beitman BD: The relation between alcohol problems and the anxiety disorders. Am J Psychiatry 1990;147:685–695.

Lader M: The nature of anxiety. Br J Psychiatry 1972;121:481–491.

Leckman JF, Merikangas KR, Pauls DL, Weissman MM, Prusoff BA, Kidd KK: Anxiety disorders and depression: Contradiction between family study data and DSM-III convention. Am J Psychiatry 1983;140:880.

Lewis CE, Rice J, Andreasen NC, Endicott J, Hartman A: Clinical and familial correlates of alcoholism in men with unipolar major depression. Alcohol Clin Exp Res 1986;10:657–662.

Maier W, Merikangas KR: Co-occurrence and co-transmission of affective disorders, anxiety disorders and alcoholism in families. Br J Psychiatry 1996;168(suppl 30):93–100.

Marks I, Lader M: Anxiety states (anxiety neurosis): A review. J Nerv Ment Dis 1978;156:3–18.

Meller WH, Rinehart R, Cadoret RJ, Troughton E: Specific familial transmission in substance abuse. Int J Addict 1988;23:1029–1039.

Merikangas KR, Gelernter CS: Comorbidity for alcoholism and depression. Psychiatr Clin North Am 1990;13:613–632.

Merikangas KR, Leckman JF, Prusoff BA, Pauls DL, Weissman MM: Familial transmission of depression and alcoholism. Arch Gen Psychiatry 1985;42:367–372.

Merikangas KR, Risch NJ, Weissman MM: Comorbidity, and co-transmission of alcoholism, anxiety and depression. Psychol Med 1994;24:69–80.

Merikangas KR, Stevens DE, Fenton B, Stolar M, O'Malley S, Woods SW, Risch N: Comorbidity and familial transmission of alcoholism and anxiety disorders. Psychol Med 1998;28:773–788.

Mirin SM, Weiss RD, Griffin ML, Michael JL: Psychopathology in drug abusers and their families. Compr Psychiatry 1991;32:36–51.

Mirin SM, Weiss RD, Michael J, Griffin ML: Psychopathology in substance abusers: Diagnosis and treatment. Am J Drug Alcohol Abuse 1988;14:139–157.

Mirin SM, Weiss RD, Sollogub A, Michael J: Psychopathology in the families of drug abusers; in Mirin SM (ed): Substance Abuse and Psychopathology. Washington, American Psychiatric Press, 1984, pp 80–106.

Mullaney JA, Trippett C: Alcohol dependence and phobias: Clinical description and relevance. Br J Psychiatry 1979;135:565–573.

Müller R: Zur Epidemiologie des Konsums legaler und illegaler Drogen in der Schweiz. Ther Umschau/ Rev Thér 1982;8:Heft 8.

Munjack DJ, Moss HB: Affective disorder and alcoholism in families of agoraphobics. Arch Gen Psychiatry 1981;38:868–871.

Nelson E, Rice J, Rochberg N, Endicott J, Coryell W, Akiskal HS: Affective illness in family members and matched controls. Acta Psychiatr Scand 1995;91:146–151.

Noyes R Jr, Clancy J, Crowe R, Hoenk RP, Slymen DJ: The familial prevalence of anxiety neurosis. Arch Gen Psychiatry 1978;35:1057–1074.

Nunes EV, Quitkin FM, Klein DF: Psychiatric diagnosis in cocaine abuse. Psychiatry Res 1989;8:105–114.

Pharma Information: Das Gesundheitswesen in der Schweiz: Leistungen, Kosten, Preise. Basel, 1996.

Preisig M, Merikangas KR: Comorbidity and co-transmission of drug abuse and alcoholism; in Symp Comorbidity in Families: Mechanisms and Treatment. Am Psychiatr Assoc Meet, New York City, May 1996.

Quitkin FM, Rifkin A, Kaplan J, Klein DF: Phobic anxiety syndrome complicated by drug dependence and addiction. Arch Gen Psychiatry 1972;45:1023–1031.

Regier DA,, Farmer ME, Rae DS, Locke BZ, Keith SJ, Judd LL, Goodwin FK: Comorbidity of mental disorders with alcohol and other drug abuse: Results from the Epidemiologic Catchment Area study. JAMA 1990;264:2511–2518.

Rehm J: Konsumformen und Verbreitung illegaler Drogen in der Schweiz; in Fahrenkrug H, Rehm J, Müller R, Klingemann H,Linder R (eds): Illegale Drogen in der Schweiz 1990–1993. Zurich; Seismo, 1995.

Reuband KH: Drug use and drug policy in Western Europe. Eur Addict Res 1995;1:32–41.

Roelofs SM: Hyperventilation, anxiety, craving for alcohol: A subacute alcohol withdrawal syndrome. Alcohol 1985;2:501–505.

Ross HE, Glaser FB, Germanson T: The prevalence of psychiatric disorders in patients with alcohol and other drug problems. Arch Gen Psychiatry 1988;45:1023–1031.

Rounsaville B: The role of psychopathology in the familial transmission of drug abuse. NIDA Res Monogr 1988;89:108–119.

Rounsaville BJ, Anton SF, Caroll K, Budde D, Prusoff BA, Gawin F: Psychiatric diagnosis of treatment-seeking cocaine abusers. Arch Gen Psychiatry 1991;48:43–51.

Rounsaville BJ, Weissman MM, Kleber H, Wilber C: Heterogeneity of psychiatric diagnosis in treated opiate addicts. Arch Gen Psychiatry 1982;128:1132–1136.

Schick MT, Alberto YL: Epidemiologische Analyse der Drogentodesfälle in der Schweiz 1990–1993 unter Einbezug der Jahre 1987–1989: Schlussbericht zuhanden des Bundesamtes für Gesundheit. Bern, Institut für Sozial- und Präventivmedizin de Universität Bern, 1994.

Schuckit MA: The clinical implications of primary diagnostic groupings among alcoholics. Arch Gen Psychiatry 1985;42:1043–1049.

Schuckit MA, Irwin M, Brown SA: The history of anxiety symptoms among 171 primary alcoholics. J Stud Alcohol 1990;51:34–41.

Smail P, Stockwell T, Canter S, Hodgson R: Alcohol dependence and phobic anxiety states. I. A prevalence study. Br J Psychiatry 1984;144:53–57.

Stabenau JR: Is the risk for substance abuse unitary? J Nerv Ment Dis 1992;180:583–588.

Stockwell T, Smail P, Hodgson R, Canter S: Alcohol dependence and phobic anxiety states. II. A retrospective study. Br J Psychiary 1984;144:58–63.

Weiss KJ, Rosenberg DJ: Prevalence of anxiety disorder among alcoholics. J Clin Psychiatry 1985;46:3–5.

Weiss RD, Mirin SM, Michael JL, Sollogub AC: Psychopathology in chronic cocaine abusers. Am J Drug Alcohol Abuse 1986;12:17–29.

Weissman MM, Myers JK: Clinical depression in alcoholism. Am J Psychiatry 1980;137:372–373.

Winokur G, Cook B, Liskow B, Fowler R: Alcoholism in manic depressive (bipolar) patients. J Stud Alcohol 1993;54:574–576.

Winokur G, Coryell W: Familial alcoholism in primary unipolar depressive disorder. Am J Psychiatry 1991;148:184–188.

Winokur G, Rimmr J, Reich T: Alcoholism IV. Is there more than one type of alcoholism? Br J Psychiatry 1971;118:525–531.

Wittchen HU, Essau CA, von Zerssen D, Krieg JC, Zaudig M: Lifetime and six-month prevalence of mental disorders in the Munich Follow-up Study. Eur Arch Psychiatry Clin Neurosci 1992;241:247–258.

Wittchen HU, Perkonigg A, Reed V: Comorbidity of mental disorders and substance use disorders. Eur Addict Res 1996;2:36–47.

Woodruff RH, Guze SB, Clayton PJ: Anxiety neurosis among psychiatric outpatients. Compr Psychiatry 1972;13:165–170.

Dr. Martin Preisig, Département universitaire de psychiatrie adulte (DUPA),
Unité de recherche en épidémiologie et psychopathologie,
Route de Cery, CH–1008 Prilly-Lausanne (Switzerland)
Tel. +41 21 643 61 11, Fax +41 21 643 62 76, E-Mail martin.preisig@inst.hospvd.ch

Ladewig D (ed): Basic and Clinical Science of Substance Related Disorders.
Bibl Psychiatr. Basel, Karger, 1999, No 168, pp 40–44

·······················

From Neuroscience to Psychoscience

The Integration of Drug Therapy and Psychotherapy into a Coordinated Dependency Management Project

J. Besson

Substance Abuse Division, Lausanne University, Lausanne, Switzerland

Clinicians working in the dependency field are living exciting times as witnesses to an ever-increasing number of discoveries on the relationships between psychoactive substances and the brain. Even if most of these new findings have come from animal studies, they shed fresh light on day-to-day clinical experience. In particular, the advances in the neurosciences herald new and highly promising prospects in pharmacology.

A cloud over these developments is the fact that not only is the number of patients dependent on psychoactive substances very great but that a fair proportion slip through the health system net. Even when they do gain access to healthcare institutions providing psychosocial support, there is still some way to go before their rehabilitation programs reflect the advances in fundamental research. Indeed, there is often a great divide between medicine on the one hand and psychotherapy and psychosocial intervention on the other; they can be worlds apart, and at times in ideological conflict. Furthermore, in Switzerland, convergence is not encouraged by the welfare and health insurance systems. A complicating factor is that public opinion, the media and politicians engage in slanging matches over the handling of the dependency problem, often in sloganistic terms that tar all treatment solutions with the same brush instead of incorporating them into a program that offers specific solutions for specific types of patients. On an ethical level, clinicians have a professional and moral duty to ensure that their most underprivileged patient on the street benefits from the results of research.

This report describes the approach we have adopted in the Substance Abuse Division in Lausanne. A point to note at the outset is that neuroscience enjoys full scientific status whereas the psychosocial sciences ('psychoscience')

have yet to find a place between the exact and human sciences. For clinicians, it is essential to integrate neuroscience and psychoscience if we are to advance clinical research and develop a coordinated chain of care. I shall give some examples from our Lausanne experience illustrating the institutional facilities and lines of clinical research which aim to meet these objectives.

Neuroscience vs. Psychoscience

Neuroscience covers a constellation of sciences orbiting the central nervous system, from molecular biology to epidemiology, encompassing genetics, neurophysiology, psychopharmacology, and also imaging. The scientific status of all these disciplines is undisputed, and their methodologies are well-established: they belong wholly to the world of research-based natural science.

Psychoscience for its part covers a constellation of approaches to mental life, from individual psychotherapy in all its forms to interventions in the economic, political or cultural spheres, via networks of psychosocial approaches, work within the community and other forms of social therapy. Their scientific status is less clear-cut; their research methods differ from those in the natural sciences. Psychoscience is human science in all its complexity. Its scientific status can only be clarified by advancing research-based knowledge within its field.

How to Advance Clinical Dependency Research

Clinical research is at a crossroads between the natural and human sciences. It is ideally placed to mesh these two worldviews and enhance the efficacy of therapeutic intervention. Our first job is better to define our methods in clinical dependency research.

We must improve our definition of the patient using ICD-10 or DSM-IV diagnostic criteria, taking all psychiatric and somatic comorbidity into account. We must use validated and standardized psychometric scales for all quantitative variables, e.g. the Addiction Severity Index (ASI), the Recovery Attitude and Treatment Evaluator (RAATE), the Obsessive-Compulsive Drinking Scale (OCDS) and the Short Form (SF) 36. We need to specify important contributors to patients' lives, such as personality structure and contextual crisis, and itemize the resources available to them.

We must improve our definition of therapeutic intervention beginning at the pharmacological level, by defining whether the pharmacotherapy is prescribed in order to wean a patient off a drug of abuse, to treat comorbidity, to substitute for – or dissuade from – a drug of abuse or, as in the case of a new entity, to decrease craving directly. Psychotherapeutic intervention must be described and specified, and maximally standardized. Intervention on the patient's context must also be recorded, in particular when it involves the family and immediate circle, but also the healthcare system (e.g. support for the family doctor).

We must also be clearer about what kind of results we expect. Much misunderstanding over the results of research arises from confusion as to the purpose of intervention. Clinical research must therefore be placed within its context, above all with respect to the concept of a therapeutic intervention threshold (e.g. are we dealing with a risk reduction program, or on the contrary a relapse prevention program?). The results should also be measured against the achievement of objectives incorporated in a written pretreatment contract. Lastly, if the intended objectives have not been met, there must be a fail-safe program of preplanned algorithms to maintain patients within the therapeutic network at a less demanding level.

This definition of integrated clinical research incorporates the bio-psycho-social aspects of dependency treatments with the twin aim of enhancing interventional efficacy and introducing the conditions of possibility for quality assurance.

How to Improve the Therapeutic Chain

A major task in global interventions and integrated clinical research is to overcome the 'medical' vs. 'social' divide. Our experience of opening a multidisciplinary reception and ambulatory treatment center for drug abusers in the Lausanne area may be instructive in this context. We opened the St. Martin Center in 1996 after reviewing the healthcare system's failings with the aim of creating an institution that would incorporate all the requirements for a global approach:
- The reception capability is paramount, with a minimum of barriers to treatment, even if it means anonymous interviews or discussing only partial aspects of treatment.
- The Center has developed a working relationship with the other healthcare and support institutions. A plainclothes MD maintains contact two evenings a week with the street scene.
- The multidisciplinary team comprises some 15 individuals including MDs (internists and psychiatrists), psychologists, general and psychiatric nurses, social workers, youth workers, and secretaries with dependency training. The idea is to provide a therapeutic facility along the lines of one-stop shopping, using the synergy that comes from maximal team coordination,

i.e. to offer clinical medicine, psychiatry, and/or social intervention all within the same facility.
- The St. Martin Center provides primary care before referring patients to other points within the network, in particular to members of the Vaud Association of Physicians Concerned about Drug Dependency (AVMCT).
- The Center supports local family doctors with advice, particularly on psychiatric problems. It offers a hotline, crisis intervention in the event of complications in the community methadone program, and postgraduate training in dependency issues.
- The St. Martin Center also offers support to rehabilitation programs with brief targeted medical interventions, without seeking to compete with their work.
- The Center runs training, teaching and research programs with and for fellow professionals.

Two Illustrations

Two examples of clinical research from the Lausanne experience may help to show how psychoscience can mesh with neuroscience.

Alcohol Dependency
Here is an example of how psychoscience provided an objective complement to psychopharmacology. When our group was approached to set up a double-blind controlled efficacy study of acamprosate vs. placebo, we thought it might be interesting for the study to incorporate the grass-root practice in our locality, i.e. the regular use of Antabus courses in the healthcare system. In the scientific literature Antabus may not have proved pharmacologically effective when used alone in self-administration, but there is a current revival of interest in the drug when incorporated into shared-care programs and cognitive-behavioral therapies. We therefore performed a controlled study of acamprosate vs. placebo, stratified for disulfiram where patients requested it. The results were extremely interesting: acamprosate outperformed placebo in all scenarios, but we found an unmistakably synergistic effect in the patients taking both substances. The synergy was not simple pharmacology but a psychotherapeutic complement to the psychopharmacological effect of acamprosate. Obviously the patients with or without disulfiram were not comparable, since those asking for a course of disulfiram were more motivated. In both cases, patients were improved by acamprosate. This type of study shows the avenue to follow in integrated clinical research that incorporates psychoscience, neuroscience and reality on the ground.

Drug Dependency

Now let us see how laboratory neuroscience added a new dimension to the methadone program. In the Department of Adult Psychiatry at Lausanne University, the Biochemistry Unit is working on methadone metabolism. It has taken part in basic research showing that methadone metabolism is distributed unequally in the general population, 5% of whom are slow metabolizers and 5% ultrafast metabolizers. This input from pharmacogenetics proved highly relevant to our analysis of treatment resistance in methadone programs. It helped in adjusting individual doses, and in training family doctors accordingly. It has even been hypothesized that we shall find a number of ultrafast methadone metabolizers among habitual dropouts from heroin programs (one such study is currently running in Switzerland).

Prospects and Conclusions

It can thus be seen that there is considerable heterogeneity among patients with psychoactive substance dependency. The correlate is to offer therapy which is correspondingly heterogeneous. This implies developing different levels of care, to be distributed between various groups of health system and social work professionals who would otherwise become dispersed unless coordinated into a coherent chain of therapy. One way to work towards this goal is to undertake integrated clinical research that draws upon neuroscience, psychoscience, and reality on the ground. The worlds of medicine and social intervention must get to know one other and plan their efforts in unison; a program of continuing education by and for the respective professionals will help to make this possible. Such an operation is complex, and structured quality assurance auditing will be mandatory to ensure that it is effective. The question guiding our future work then becomes the following: what is the right treatment for the right patient at the right time?

Dr. Jacques Besson, Département universitaire de psychiatrie adulte (DUPA),
Direction des Dépendances, Centre Saint Martin,
Rue St. Martin 7, CH–1003 Lausanne (Switzerland)
Tel. +41 21 316 16 01, Fax +41 21 316 16 36, E-Mail jacques.besson@inst-hospvd.ch

Ladewig D (ed): Basic and Clinical Science of Substance Related Disorders.
Bibl Psychiatr. Basel, Karger, 1999, No 168, pp 45–48

....

Randomized Open Efficacy Study of Naltrexone vs. Acamprosate vs. Disulfiram Combined with Cognitive-Behavioral Psychotherapy in Preventing Alcohol Relapse[1]

U. von Bardeleben, H. Knoch, E. Biedert, T. Ihde, D. Ladewig

Department of Psychiatry, University of Basel, Switzerland

A standard pharmacological approach for maintaining abstinence in weaned alcoholics has been the aversive drug disulfiram, which triggers flushing, nausea, tachycardia, hypotension and dyspnea in response to alcohol ingestion. Yet, its efficacy in encouraging abstinence has been discussed controversially [1, 2]. Acamprosate and naltrexone are recently introduced alternatives which may work via partially elucidated anticraving activity. Acamprosate interacts with N-methyl-D-aspartic acid (NMDA) receptor-mediated glutamergic neurotransmission: it reduces the neural hyperexcitability of the NMDA receptors which increase in number (upregulation) under the chronic action of alcohol [3]. The significantly higher abstinence rate observed on acamprosate [4] is thought due to dampening of the craving related to conditioned withdrawal phenomena [5].

Naltrexone is an opioid antagonist reducing alcohol activation of the endogenous opioid release [5, 6] which, in the mesolimbic reward system, plays a key role in dependence diseases. Naltrexone has reduced alcohol consumption in several clinical trials [7, 8].

In nearly all pharmacotherapy studies on maintaining abstinence in weaned alcoholics, drugs have been combined with different types of short-term psychotherapy. The objective of the present study was to compare efficacy between disulfiram, acamprosate and naltrexone when each was combined with standardized short-term cognitive-behavioral psychotherapy.

[1] Supported by the Swiss National Science Foundation No. 32-43265.

Methods

The study population comprised 60 patients with alcohol dependence according to DSM-IV [9] entering the University of Basel, Department of Psychiatry, for alcohol withdrawal. 73% were men and mean age of the total sample was 44.8 ± 9.2 years. After weaning, the aims of the study were explained in detail and informed consent obtained.

Pharmacotherapy. The 60 patients were randomized to acamprosate (1,800 mg/day) or naltrexone (45 mg/day) or disulfiram (200 mg/day) on an open basis. Drug dosing was controlled.

Psychotherapy. Following inpatient treatment for several days to 2 weeks, patients participated in an outpatient manualized cognitive-behavioral group psychotherapy program for relapse prophylaxis, weekly for 12 weeks. This modified version of the group therapy program of Monti et al. [10] run by a clinical psychologist and a psychiatrist, was highly structured in form and content. It comprised the following twelve consecutive modules: (1) introduction to training in coping strategies for alcohol dependence; (2) coping with alcohol craving; (3) dealing with thoughts about alcohol; (4) general problem-solving strategies; (5) refusing alcohol (saying no); (6) dealing with seemingly insignificant decisions; (7) dealing with risk and relapse situations; (8) enforcing one's own needs; (9) dealing with criticism; (10) dealing with depressed mood; (11) dealing with anger; (12) relaxation techniques.

Laboratory Parameters. Gamma glutamyltransferase (GT) and mean corpuscular volume (MVC) were determined 4-weekly.

Statistical Analysis. Groups were compared at baseline using the chi-square test or analysis of variance (ANOVA). Results were compared between groups using the Wilcoxon-Gehan or Student's t test. A significance level of $p < 0.05$ was used in all tests.

Results

The three groups did not differ at baseline either in sociodemographics (sex, age, income, living and family conditions) or drinking behavior in the past 3 months, number of earlier withdrawals, and family stress. All three drugs were well tolerated. Diarrhea was more frequent on acamprosate and sleep disturbance more frequent on naltrexone, in neither case to the extent of causing dropout. The groups did not differ in gamma GT or MCV values. 65% of patients completed regularly the 12-week program, with no significant intergroup differences (table 1).

Although 31/60 patients (52%) admitted consuming alcohol at least once during the 12 weeks, the overall proportion of abstinent days was 90% (table 2), with no significant intergroup differences. However, the groups differed in time to first drink, which was much longer on disulfiram ($p < 0.05$); the other group comparisons were not significant. The groups did not differ in time to first relapse (defined as $< 60/40$ g alcohol/day in men/women) or in time to first serious relapse (defined as 60/40 g alcohol/day in men/women on at least 3

Table 1. Participation rates (mean ± standard deviation unless otherwise indicated)

	Disulfiram (n = 29)	Acamprosate (n = 20)	Naltrexone (n = 20)	χ^2 or ANOVA
Treatment completers, %	55	65	75	NS
Duration of observation, weeks	9.2 ± 4.0	9.6 ± 4.1	10.5 ± 3.0	NS
Psychotherapy sessions attended	7.4 ± 3.5	7.8 ± 3.5	6.6 ± 3.2	NS

Table 2. Treatment results (median, or mean ± standard deviation)

	Disulfiram (D)	Acamprosate (A)	Naltrexone (N)	p < 0.05 D vs. A	D vs. N	A vs. N
Abstinence days, %	93.3 ± 16.6	93.3 ± 15.2	85.9 ± 20.2	NS	NS	NS
Time to first drink, weeks	> 12	6	10	0.02*	0.04*	NS
Time to first relapse, weeks (> 60/40 g alcohol in men/women)	> 12	9	> 12	NS	NS	NS
Time to first serious relapse (> 60/40 g alcohol in men/women over 3 days)	> 12	> 12	> 12	NS	NS	NS
Alcohol/day, g	165.1 ± 96.6	85.7 ± 55.5	58.9 ± 43.4	0.04**	0.02**	NS

* Wilcoxon-Gehan test; ** t test.

successive days). However, analysis of the amounts drunk showed a far higher intake on a drinking day in the disulfiram group (165.1 ± 96.6 g) than with naltrexone (85.7 ± 55.5 g) or acamprosate (58.9 ± 43.4 g).

Attendance of the group psychotherapy sessions was 66%. Semistructured survey revealed that 60% of patients considered they had acquired new insight into their problem and a readiness for behavioral change. 55% ascribed their approval of the program as due to its contextual and formal structure.

Discussion

A 65% therapy completion rate and a 90% overall proportion of abstinent days are both high figures in dependency study terms and can be presumed due to the combined effect of the drugs and cognitive-behavioral group therapy. The population was too small to draw more detailed conclusions. The three drugs were similarly effective if abstinence is defined as time to first relapse rather than as time to first drink. On disulfiram, the number of abstinent days during the 12 weeks was the same as in the other two groups, but time to first drink was longest; however, the daily amount consumed during relapse was also the highest, possibly due to the recognized abstinence-violation effect which could have been most marked in this group.

The 66% attendance rate at the psychotherapy session was also a satisfactory approval rating in a dependency study, and was supposed by patients' responses to the semistructured survey. When combined with the relatively low 35% dropout rate during the study, these figures support the concept of a combination of psychotherapy and pharmacotherapy in the outpatient management of alcohol dependence.

References

1 Fuller RK, Branchey L, Brightwell DR, Derman RM, Emrick CD, Iber FL, James KE, Lacoursiere RB, Lee KK, Lowenstam I: Disulfiram treatment of alcoholism: A Veterans Administration cooperative study. JAMA 1986;256:1449–1455.
2 Chick J, Gough K, Falkowski W, Kershaw P, Hore B, Mehta B, Ritson B, Ropner R, Torley D: Disulfiram treatment of alcoholism. Br J Psychiatry 1992;162:84–89.
3 Zieglgänsberger W, Hauser C, Wetzel C, Putzke J, Siggins GR, Spanagel R: Actions of acamprosate on neurons of the central nervous system; in Soyka M (ed): Acamprosate in Relapse Prevention of Alcoholism. Heidelberg, Springer, 1996, pp 65–70.
4 Sass H, Soyka M, Mann K, Zieglgänsberger W: Relapse prevention by acamprosate: Results from a placebo-controlled study on alcohol dependence. Arch Gen Psychiatry 1996;53:673–680.
5 Spanagel R, Zieglgänsberger W: Anticraving compounds for ethanol: New pharmacological tools to study addictive process. Trends Pharmacol Sci 1997;18:54–59.
6 Herz A: Endogenous opioid systems and alcohol addiction. Psychopharmacology 1997;129:99–111.
7 Volpicelli JR, Rhines KC, Rhines JS, Volpicelli LA, Alterman Al, O'Brien CP: Naltrexone and alcohol dependence: Role of subject compliance. Arch Gen Psychiatry 1997;54:737–742.
8 O'Malley S, Jaffe AJ, Change G, Schottenfeld RS, Meyer RE, Rounsaville B: Naltrexone and coping skills therapy for alcohol dependence. Arch Gen Psychiatry 1992;49:881–887.
9 American Psychiatric Association: Diagnostic and Statistical Manual of Mental Disorders, ed 4. Washington, American Psychiatric Association, 1994.
10 Monti PM, Abrams DB, Kadden RM, Cooney NL: Treating Alcohol Dependence: A Coping Skill Training Guide. New York, Guilford Press, 1989.

Prof. Dr. D. Ladewig, Department of Psychiatry, University of Basel,
Wilhelm Klein-Strasse 27, CH–4025 Basel (Switzerland)
Tel. +41 61 325 51 37, Fax +41 61 325 55 83, E-Mail dieter.ladewig@pukbasel.ch

Ladewig D (ed): Basic and Clinical Science of Substance Related Disorders.
Bibl Psychiatr. Basel, Karger, 1999, No 168, pp 49–55

....

Clinical Addiction Research between Health Care Responsibility and Basic Research

D. Ladewig

Department of Psychiatry, University of Basel, Switzerland

The use of psychotropic substances has increased worldwide, a fact with major health policy implications given the now considerable attendant socio-economic cost. The public reacts in differing ways, often emotionally, with shock and fear, or by trivializing the issue. Opioid or cocaine use and the risk of AIDS provoke fear. The alleged cardioprotective effect of alcoholic drinks diverts attention from the dangers of harmful use. While the seventies and eighties saw physicians becoming increasingly restrictive in their attitude to narcotic analgesics, and eventually reluctant to prescribe them at all, there is now again a growing tendency to use opioids for the treatment of severe pain. And while nicotine is today generally held to be harmful, recent smoking cessation studies show that occasional patients become chronically depressed and require treatment following nicotine withdrawal. Consequently, any assessment of the risks and benefits of psychotropic substances such as alcohol, nicotine, cannabis, opioids, cocaine, amphetamines and benzodiazepines must consider a wide variety of factors, whose importance varies at different historical moments. The medical use of psychotropic substances must therefore be subjected to constant critical scrutiny and reevaluation [Pletscher and Ladewig, 1994]. Below I outline some aspects of clinical addiction research, as I have observed it over the past 30 years.

Dependence Terminology

The term 'dependence' [Eddy, 1955] represented a milestone in the linguistic understanding of addictive behavior, determining the development of modern diagnostics in the ICD and DSM. Dependence was operationalized by clinical criteria and described according to classes of substance with differing clinical actions. Disregarded, though, were questions on the etiology, development and course of dependence syndromes, and especially on the reversibility of addictive behavior. If dependence is the result of a continuum from use to dependence, then there must also be a 'reverse continuum', or remissions. The discussion about the 'point of no return', as against the controlled use by addicts of alcohol or even heroin, illustrates the field of conflict and the broadness of the spectrum of 'dependence'. If dependences are today understood in a biopsychosocial context, then biological [Spanagel, this vol.] and psychosocial issues – e.g. vulnerability [Wittchen, this vol.] – must be taken into account.

Opinions differ on which and how many *criteria* are to be used in diagnosing dependence. The inclusion of criteria based on abstinence symptoms accords with a restrictive viewpoint, and traditionally that of the clinician. Their exclusion reflects an emphasis on the psychosocial dimension, with enhanced importance attached to the diagnosis 'abuse' or 'harmful use'. In adolescents at risk of addiction, multimorbid psychiatric patients or members of marginalized social groups, such as immigrants, any dependence disorder is manifested primarily in psychosocial terms, including in psychological dependence. A dependence syndrome or substance abuse is then often offered as a second or third diagnosis together with another psychiatric diagnosis. Physical dependence is of secondary importance compared with the subjective desire for substance use – as an attempt to cope with intra- or interpersonal crises.

Dependences lead to *secondary disorders*, which vary with substance type. These are well researched in the case of alcohol dependence, but poorly so in opioid, cannabis or cocaine dependence, reflecting their less frequent occurrence. In the past this continually led to a dangerous polarization between 'legal' addictive substances – principally alcohol – that cause somatic damage and 'illegal' drugs, such as opioids, cocaine or cannabis, whose use does comparatively little physical harm. Brain research has not only enlarged our understanding of alcohol-induced deficits but revealed new avenues for investigating the effects and possible long-term consequences of opioids and cocaine.

The last few years have witnessed an exponential increase in our knowledge of gene-environment interaction and its effects on the brain. In particular, family, twin and adoption studies suggest that substance abuse and dependence have a genetic component. Vulnerability to alcohol dependence is polygenically determined and shows marked interindividual variation. Alcohol-related factors are, for example, alcohol preference, sensitivity and tolerance, which are based in turn on hereditary factors and in some cases neurotransmission abnormalities. Low activity of the central serotonin system has been proposed as a genetically controlled vulnerability factor for the development of alcohol dependence, with impulsive-aggressive behavior and early onset of abuse defining a subtype of alcoholic with a pronounced genetic predisposition to alcohol dependence [Schuckit, 1992; Merikangas et al., 1994; Maier, 1996].

In contrast to alcohol dependence, with possible subgroups and links to other psychiatric syndromes, such as anxiety disorders, drug – and especially opioid – users have been relatively poorly studied with regard to genetic vulnerability. The twin studies undertaken to date support the hypothesis of genetic factors in the development of drug abuse or drug problems [Pickens and Svikis, 1991; Jang et al., 1995]. A recent adoption study [Cadoret et al., 1995] produced evidence that a diagnosis of 'antisocial personality disorder' in one parent leads to aggressiveness, antisocial personality disorder and ultimately drug problems in the adopted child.

The relationship between *psychiatry* and dependence disorders was long characterized by ambivalence. In recent times increasing attention has been paid to the issue of *comorbidity*, i.e. the presence of coexisting psychiatric diseases. Comorbid patients display worse compliance, greater morbidity and mortality risks and a higher risk of social disintegration and criminality. Comorbid disorders are increased in all forms of dependence, including in opioid users and addicts. In the case of personality disorders, quoted prevalences range from 30 to 90%, depending on study population, diagnostic algorithm employed and time window [Clerici and Carta, 1996]. Affective and anxiety disorders must be expected in 20–60% of drug-dependent patients, as against schizophreniform disorders in 0–20% [Galanter and Castaneda, 1991].

Concern with addiction problems has a certain tradition in Swiss psychiatry, which is one factor behind the current search for new approaches, for example in maintenance medications [Ladewig, 1990] or recently in the national PROVE projects [Uchtenhagen et al., 1997]. In the completed PROVE projects, attention was focused not only on new dosage forms but also for the first time on heroin as a new maintenance substance.

With the dramatic growth of the drug scene in European cities in the 1980s, and prompted in particular by HIV spread and the increasing destitution of the most severely addicted users, there developed in Switzerland a practice of dispensing syringes, expanding methadone maintenance programs, and establishing street centers (Gassenzimmer), night shelters and integrated emergency medical care. The facilities were made as decentralized and accessible as possible with the aim of identifying drug addicts at an early stage and providing them with effective aids to survival. These efforts succeeded in delimiting the Swiss drug scene and stabilizing the health of many drug addicts, thereby stemming the growing problem.

In addition, psychiatry strives for a cause-oriented approach in both treatment and prevention. In principle, addiction prevention and addiction treatment must always be viewed in the context of 'substance supply and demand'. Historically, the supply or accessibility of drugs implied prohibition, or all restrictive measures imposed by law and enforced by criminal prosecution. In keeping with its self-image and task, psychiatry has tended to concentrate on the demand side. In the past this implied a certain primacy for abstinence-oriented treatment strategies. This basic approach dominates the field of alcoholism. The use of so-called anticraving substances can today help a significant proportion of patients to reduce their harmful alcohol consumption [von Bardeleben et al., this vol.].

Substance-Specific Research

The use of *cannabis* products is today generally viewed in a sociocultural context. Although the toxic effects of the active agents are undisputed, conventional use rarely leads to intoxications, psychotic reactions or abstinence syndromes requiring therapeutic intervention. Whereas interest previously focused on the immediate effect of the substance, for example in relation to driving behavior [Kielholz et al., 1973], cannabis use in drug-dependent and psychiatric patients is today more likely to provoke questions on the implications of concomitant use, in other words, interactions of all neuroleptic or antidepressant medications with cannabis and, where relevant, methadone.

Despite intensive research into the mechanisms of action of *cocaine*, it has not yet proved possible to develop effective pharmacotherapeutic strategies for cocaine dependence treatment or relapse prevention [Kleber, 1995; O'Brien, 1996]. Among cocaine users there appears to be a clinically particularly relevant group distinguished from other users by pronounced sensation seeking, severe psychosocial impairment, intensive use, tendency to polysubstance abuse, and positive (family) history of antisocial personality disorder and attention deficit hyperactivity disorder [Ball et al., 1994]. A special problem is that of cocaine use by methadone-maintained heroin addicts. Here again a favored pharmacotherapeutic strategy has yet to emerge, despite numerous studies.

Benzodiazepines are today firmly established in the medical arsenal. They are important drugs in many disorders and indispensable especially to the anesthetist, psychiatrist and general practitioner. The dependence potential of benzodiazepines is well known [Ladewig, 1984]. Unfortunately, research into the benefit-risk ratio of long-term benzodiazepine use has received no major fresh impetus in recent years. Given the wide use and effectiveness of these drugs, problems inevitably arise when they are used in high-risk populations and for inappropriate indications. This applies in particular to elderly patients and drug addicts, in whom concomitant use leads to polydependence, as well as delirium, twilight states and states with increased danger to self and others. The frequently observed preference for certain benzodiazepines, such as flunitrazepam, has still to be adequately explained.

Opioids remain important strong analgesics and are used as such. A basic therapeutic approach has also crystallized with regard to maintenance of opioid addicts. The practice varies from one country to another but shows a clear trend, including towards the involvement of general practitioners. With increased use of opioids in maintenance treatment, our knowledge of effects and side effects has also grown. Our own observations on the occurrence of epileptiform disorders in the Heroin Prescription project conducted in Basel by the University Department of Psychiatry prompted EEG and later infrared spectroscopic studies at the time of heroin administration. The latter showed that cortical hemoglobin oxygenation is reduced after heroin exposure [Stohler et al., this vol.; Hock et al., 1998]. The reason for this fall in oxygen saturation remains unclear; modifying factors include distribution rate, dosage and additive effects of other substances. These observations show that patient care cannot be the sole consideration in maintenance treatment. To assure the quality of these treatments, it is also necessary to examine biological questions, whether on the 'rush effect' or certain side effects. This is not to belittle the significance of maintenance treatments, including with heroin. The fundamentally positive effects of mortality reduction and decriminalization are of central importance in harm reduction and assuring the survival of opioid addicts. Research is also necessary in the psychosocial sphere. What patients on maintenance programs require additional psychotherapeutic and perhaps pharmacotherapeutic support? Assuring the future quality of these treatments will not be possible without further research.

The previous restriction to methadone-based maintenance treatment has been loosened with the Heroin Prescription projects (PROVE). Apart from this, there appear to be good arguments for broadening the spectrum of maintenance medications. The partial agonist/antagonist buprenorphine [Ling et al., 1996; Strain et al., 1994] has recently been proposed as a promising alternative to methadone.

The increased range of treatment options for opioid addicts represents an important addition to the earlier – exclusively nonpharmacotherapeutic – methods. It should be remembered that the long-term prognosis for opioid addicts is not as bad as often assumed. In longitudinal studies carried out in Switzerland in the eighties in the context of a national research program on social integration, nearly 40% of drug addicts had achieved opiate abstinence after 5 years of observation [Ladewig and Graw, 1985, 1987].

In the area of *alcohol* research, we find a wealth of new biological approaches. Clinical epidemiology is increasingly studying vulnerability traits in families with an increased occurrence of dependence disorders and comorbid psychiatric syndromes. In the field of treatment research, preliminary experience with anticraving substances has raised new hopes of broadening the range of options for helping alcoholics. Here it has been clear from the outset that only well-integrated treatments giving due attention to cognitive and psychosocial aspects can produce success.

Besides *substance-specific* research issues, attention must today also be paid to common aspects of addiction development and treatment, regardless of substance. Such general features of addiction have, for example, been identified for alcohol, opiate and amphetamine use patterns by behavioral pharmacology studies in animals. An overarching perspective also commends itself to the clinician, since most addicts treated today are polysubstance abusers [Ladewig and Schröter, 1990]. In this area there have been great changes over the years. Until into the seventies, for example, phenacetin misuse was viewed in Switzerland as an important psychiatric, sociomedical and nephrological problem [Kielholz and Ladewig, 1977; Ladewig, 1993].

The field of intervention and health care research is increasingly focusing on the common needs of alcohol- and drug-dependent individuals. Strict segregation has historical significance and makes sense in the clinical setting, e.g. in withdrawal treatments.

Clinical addiction research in psychiatry has slowly gained a foothold in a number of European countries in the last few years. In particular, through its 'Addiction Research' grant program, the German Ministry of Education, Science, Research and Technology has made available funds for basic research, which should eventually lead to advances in clinical research [Ladewig, 1997]. A key aim of this program is collaborative research, in other words, the creation of regional research structures. This model should also attract interest in other European countries and help to overcome deficits in clinical addiction research. What is unfortunately sorely lacking is internationally coordinated sponsorship of new academic talent. Bodies corresponding to the National Institute on Drug Abuse (NIDA) in the United States represent the first steps in this direction. European countries will have to seek ways and means of creating the structural framework for sponsoring young researchers.

References

Ball SA, Carroll KM, Rounsaville BJ: Sensation seeking, substance abuse, and psychopathology in treatment-seeking and community cocaine abusers. J Consult Clin Psychol 1994;62:1053–1057.

Cadoret RJ, Yates WR, Troughton E, Woolsworth G, Stewart MA: Adoption study demonstrating two genetic pathways to drug abuse. Arch Gen Psychiatry 1995;52:42–52.

Clerici M, Carta I: Personality disorders among psychoactive substance users. Eur Addict Res 1996;2: 147–155.

Eddy NB: The phenomena of tolerance; in Sevag MG, Reid RD, Reynolds OE (eds): Origins of Resistance to Toxic Agents. New York, Academic Press, 1955, pp 223–243.

Galanter M, Castaneda R: Studies of prevalence of dual diagnosis in psychiatric practice, in Gold MS, Slyby AE (eds): Dual Diagnosis in Substance Abuse. New York, Dekker, 1991.

Hock C, Störmer R, Dürstcler K, Müller-Spahn F, Ladewig D, Stohler R: Heroin-induced deoxygenation of cerebral hemoglobin: Monitoring by means of near-infrared spectroscopy. Ann Neurol, 1998

Jang KL, Livesley WJ, Vernon PA: Alcohol and drug problems: A multivariate behavioral genetic analysis of comorbidity. Addiction 1995;90:1213–1221.

Kielholz P, Ladewig D: Abuse of non-narcotic analgesics; in Martin WR (ed): Handbook of Experimental Pharmacology. Heidelberg, Springer, 1977, pp 667–672.

Kielholz P, Hobi V, Ladewig D, Miest P, Richter R: An experimental investigation about the effect of Cannabis on car driving behavior. Pharmakopsychiatrie 1973;6:91–103.

Kleber HD: Pharmacotherapy, current and potential, for the treatment of cocaine dependence. Clin Neuropharmacol 1995;18(suppl 1):96–109.

Ladewig D: Dependence liability of the benzodiazepines. Drug Alcohol Depend 1984;13:139–149.

Ladewig D: Opiate maintenance and abstinence: Attidues, treatment modalities and outcome. Drug Alcohol Depend 1990;25:245–250.

Ladewig D: The abuse of non-narcotic analgesics; in Stewart JH (ed): Analgesic NSAID-Induced Kidney Disease. Oxford Monogr Clin Nephrol, Oxford Medical Publications. Oxford, University Press, 1993, pp 48–57.

Ladewig D: BMBF-Förderschwerpunkt Suchtforschung: Bericht über das Statusseminar am 27./28. November 1997 in Bad Honnef. Sucht 1997;43:156–162.

Ladewig D, Graw P: Entwicklungen bei Drogenabhängigkeit. Weinheim, Belz, 1985.

Ladewig D, Graw P: Entwicklungsverläufe Opiatabhängiger über 6 Jahre (1979 bis 1985). Soz Präventivmed 1987;32:127–132.

Ladewig D, Schroeter U: Drug dependence in patients in psychiatric hospitals in Switzerland. Pharmacopsychiatry 1990;4:182–186.

Ling W, Wesson DR, Charuvastra C, Klett CJ: A controlled trial comparing buprenorphine and methadone maintenance in opioid dependence. Arch Gen Psychiatry 1996;53:401–407.

Maier W: Genetik von Alkoholabusus und Alkoholabhängigkeit; in Mann K, Buchkremer G (eds): Sucht, Grundlagen, Diagnostik, Therapie. Stuttgart, Fischer, 1996.

Merikangas KR, Riesch NJ, Weissmann MM: Comorbidity and co-transmission of alcoholism, anxiety and depression. Psychol Med 1994;24:69–80.

O'Brien CP: Drug addiction and drug abuse; in Hardman JG, Limbird LE, Molinoff PB, Ruddon RW, Goodman LS, Gilman A (eds): The Pharmacological Basis of Therapeutics. New York, McGraw-Hill, 1996.

Pickens RW, Svikis DS: Genetic influences in human substance abuse. J Addict Dis 1991;10:205–213.

Pletscher A, Ladewig D: 50 years of LSD, current status and perspectives of hallucinogens, incl conclusions which special regards to clinical aspects; in Pletscher A (ed): Pantenon. New York, 1994, pp 223–228.

Schuckit MA: Advances in understanding the vulnerability of alcoholism; in O'Brien CP, Jaffe JH (eds): Addictive States. New York, Raven Press, 1992, pp 93–108.

Strain EC, Stitzer ML, Liebson IA, Bigelow GE: Comparison of buprenorphine and methadone in the treatment of opioid dependence. Am J Psychiatry 1994;151:1025–1030.

Uchtenhagen A, Gutzwiller F, Dobler-Mikola A: Versuche für eine ärztliche Verschreibung von Betäubungsmitteln: Synthesebericht. Zurich, Institut für Suchtforschung (ISF), 1997.

Prof. Dr. D. Ladewig, Department of Psychiatry, University of Basel,
Wilhelm Klein-Strasse 27, CH–4025 Basel (Switzerland)
Tel. +41 61 325 51 37, Fax +41 61 325 55 83, E-Mail dieter.ladewig@pukbasel.ch

Ladewig D (ed): Basic and Clinical Science of Substance Related Disorders.
Bibl Psychiatr. Basel, Karger, 1999, No 168, pp 56–63

....

Alcoholism Today

The Rebirth of Ideologies of Individual Blame

Richard Müller

Schweizerische Fachstelle für Alkohol- und andere Drogenprobleme,
Lausanne, Switzerland

A Brief Historical Excursus

Alcohol Dependence as a Human Condition

The history of alcoholism displays close parallels to that of madness. Archaic and clerical-feudal societies viewed man as part of a numinous cosmic order rather than as a self-determining individual, and hence attached no blame to madness or alcoholism. In ancient times, alcohol use and inebriation figured in religious rites (the cult of Dionysus/Liber, the Lenaia, etc.). Seneca, the archmoralist, clearly differentiated between occasional inebriation and chronic alcoholism, a condition for which he said the individual bore no responsibility [Jellinek, 1976]. In the theocentric world view of the Middle Ages, God admittedly no longer spoke through the insane or the intoxicated, but drunkenness and mental derangement were nevertheless tolerated. While archaic thought strikingly lacked the notion of the self-conscious mind, viewing man as part of inanimate nature, feudal societies assumed the individual's total dependence on a theocentric order. Consistent with man's other-directedness, no blame attached to behaviours willed by God or otherwise associated with the divine.

'Drunkenness a Vice Not a Disease'

The groundwork for 'culpabilising' behaviours associated with alcoholism and insanity was not laid until later, during the humanist and rationalist Age of Enlightenment, when human autonomy became an operative principle of liberal ideology. Industrial society responded to the problems of madness and alcoholism by putting them out of sight and mind. The insane were marginalised, and alcoholics were stigmatised as depraved and stuck in workhouses – after all, capitalism needed sober workers [Foucault, 1961]. 'Drunkenness is a vice and not a disease' was the title of a pamphlet widely circulated in the United States and Great Britain in the 1800s. In the last century alcohol became the root of all evil, and – as a wealth of literature attests – those who drank immoderately became villains par excellence.

Alcoholism an Illness?

The situation changed dramatically towards the close of the 19th century. Socialist ideas were gaining in currency at the time and played no little part in establishing a new paradigm of human individuality. In this new view, man is conditioned by his physical and socio-political environment, and hence the scope of human responsibility is limited. Marx, for instance, speaks of man as a 'zôon politikon', a political being shaped by his surroundings. Increasingly defined as a disease, alcoholism shed much of its onus of blame and became a concern for the medical profession. The alcoholism of squalor was replaced to an ever greater extent by the alcoholism of affluence. No longer the bane of a proletariat drowning its misery in drink, alcoholism became an affliction of the elegant bourgeoisie, who found countless occasions for indulging in recreational drinking. The class connotations of drinking changed.

Drifting Back to an Ideology of Blame

And today? At a time of resurgent neoliberalism and increasing social fragmentation, when solidarity is being supplanted by a hedonistic pursuit of private happiness, we are seeing a definite drift towards new ideologies of individual blame. The notion that the costs of illness and rehabilitation should be shared is being replaced by the principle of 'causer pays'. And yet, if everybody were expected to pay for behaviour that compromised his physical or mental health, every smoker, everybody who ate improperly, worked too much or played a high-risk sport (soccer being a classic example) would have to be penalised as well. One might well wonder what claims would be left for health insurers to pay.

In view of the many social conventions that encourage drinking – not to mention the seductive advertising for tobacco products and alcoholic beverages, which has an effect even on children – it is absurd to lay the blame on society's weakest members. The extent to which social conventions promote drinking is illustrated by the frequency of alcohol consumption for different age groups in Switzerland.

As figure 1 indicates, women behave more sensibly than men (and so should be paying lower rather than higher health insurance premiums than men). Similarly, it reflects the magnitude of social pressures to drink, especially

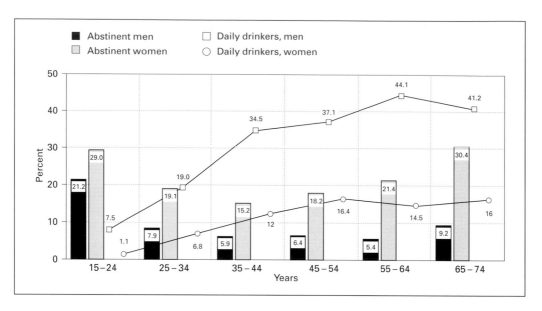

Fig. 1. Frequency of daily alcohol consumption and abstinence rates by sex and age.

among young men. The age-specific abstinence rates also show that anybody who is abstinent at age 35 is an exception to the social norm.

Vox populi, vox dei

The World Health Organization (WHO), as is well known, defines alcohol dependence unequivocally as an illness, and hence advocates social solidarity in distributing the costs of treatment. This position is embodied, for example, in the WHO's European Charter on Alcohol, to which Switzerland is a signatory. Thus the 'official' Swiss stance is also to advocate solidarity in sharing treatment costs. Is the WHO's position reflected by public opinion? Certainly the public has become much more aware of alcohol-related problems in recent years, and public attitudes to problem drinkers also bespeak a growing sensitivity. In a survey carried out in 1975, 28% of adult respondents said they knew someone with alcohol problems. By 1997 this figure had risen to 43%, despite a per capita decline in alcohol consumption over the same period. This is a clear indication of a growing public awareness.

But public perceptions of alcohol dependence remain ambivalent. While people readily concede that alcoholism is an illness, they also tend to view it as a vice. Alcoholics tend to be regarded as lazy, stubborn and withdrawn, for example. Fifteen percent of adults think alcoholics are beyond help, and a full 4% think that they do not deserve to be helped [Fahrenkrug, 1992]. These results from population surveys reflect a slight decline in social stigmatisation, but they are also indicative of a view of alcoholism as a 'chronic, hard to cure illness', a view that poses an obstacle to reintegrating alcoholics as active and productive members of the workforce. Public support for alcohol and drug testing in companies (at least in sensitive industries) also signals a defensive, watchdog mentality likely to restrict the access of controlled drinkers and former alcoholics to employment.

Alcoholism and Unemployment

The key question in regard to alcoholism and unemployment is twofold: Does unemployment cause alcohol dependence (social causation hypothesis) or does alcohol dependence cause unemployment (drift hypothesis)? These questions raise a number of methodological issues. Most of the studies done to date have been cross-sectional. Longitudinal studies, which are needed to resolve the causality question, are rare.

Of the nine panel studies carried out to date, five document a positive correlation between unemployment and alcohol consumption. Three find no correlation, and one study [Catalano et al., 1993] indicates that alcohol consumption is lower among the unemployed.

The threat of losing one's job presumably has a disciplining effect, as the sharp decline in Monday absenteeism in Switzerland suggests. People try to control their drinking and report faithfully to work simply because in a period of recession their jobs seem less secure. The drift hypothesis states that people who drink to excess gradually slip down the social ladder and ultimately lose their jobs. One longitudinal study has in fact shown that after 4 years the risk of job loss was more than twice as high among problem drinkers than among non-problem drinkers [Dooley et al., 1992]. Another longitudinal study revealed that high alcohol consumption in school leavers increased the risk of unemployment, though the same study also found that unemployment increased alcohol consumption [Janlert and Hammarström, 1992].

Perhaps the most important investigation to date in this area is a Swedish longitudinal study showing that the onset of symptoms of alcohol dependence before age 18 clearly reduces educational achievement (by a factor of 1.5), which naturally results in lower incomes and higher unemployment [Mullahy and Sindelar, 1989]. There is only one way to interpret these findings: secondary prevention is required, particularly in general practice and general hospital settings. A conclusion that certainly cannot be drawn is that alcohol abusers have no one to blame but themselves and should bear the costs of their mistakes.

Obviously the working world is bound to reflect patterns of substance abuse in the general population. Still, certain occupational cultures clearly deserve to be regarded as special risk factors beyond the individual's control. Occupations carried out in, or frequently involving, drinking situations – in the hospitality industry, say, or sales – are prime examples. (The proportion of heavy drinkers is particularly high in the building trades, among unskilled labourers, in the automotive industry and in the hospitality sector.) To blame members of these occupational groups for excessive drinking would be like blaming miners for contracting black lung disease.

Admittedly, there is no conclusive evidence about the extent to which occupational stress causes addictive behaviour; individual strategies for coping with such stress are simply too diverse for that. However, recent studies do clearly show that job dissatisfaction promotes alcohol consumption and smoking even in the early stages of working life [Frone and Windle, 1997]. Seen from this perspective, it is simply nonsense to reduce the gradual occupational impairment caused by such behaviour to a question of fault and blame.

Unemployment and Discrimination

Alcohol dependents, and former dependents, are discriminated against in the labour market. The chances of re-entering the workforce are markedly reduced for unemployed alcohol abusers, as all the statistical evidence shows. Everyone who deals with this problem is aware that discrimination reinforces alcohol use disorders and thus contributes to the development of chronic dependence. Economic recession exacerbates social discrimination against alcohol dependents and increases the tendency to blame these people for their problems. The data reveal a striking correlation between unemployment rates and the percentage of gainfully employed patients in inpatient facilities; in other words, the proportion of unemployed people being treated in rehabilitation clinics follows the ups and downs of the economic cycle (fig. 2). Not only are the unemployed overrepresented in alcohol clinics, but unemployed persons receiving treatment exhibit a higher degree of dependence. This, too, is confirmed by the SAKRAM data (table 1). If morning drinking is used as a measure of dependence, it clearly emerges that unemployed patients are more dependent than those with full-time employment.

A 2-year prospective study of 310 long-term unemployed in Norway indicates that critical alcohol consumption clearly affects the chances of alcohol

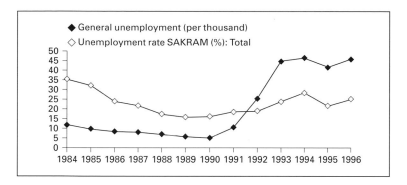

Fig. 2. Unemployment rates in the general population and among patients in alcohol clinics (SAKRAM clients).

Table 1. Unemployment and degree of dependence: time of first drink of the day prior to admission to an inpatient facility (SAKRAM 1997)

Employment status	Morning drinking, %		n
	men	women	
Full-time	40.5	35.8	293
Part-time	48.2	42.5	146
Unemployed	51.7	49.1	163

dependents finding new employment [Claussen and Aasland, 1993]. A 7-year Swiss follow-up study at alcohol clinics in German-speaking Switzerland concludes that out-of-work patients have a higher incidence of relapse and that employment increases the probability of normal completion of therapy. These findings clearly underscore the relevance of occupational integration to the course of addiction [Maffli et al., 1996].

Ability to Work as a Medical Category

Is ability to work a medical category? As a rule, inability to engage in gainful employment is defined largely in social terms, and only to a limited extent by medical criteria. There is a close but non-causal relationship between unemployment and socio-psychosomatic illnesses. These illnesses first manifest themselves clearly when they present as alcohol dependence and abuse.

Alcoholism is an illness and constitutes at least a partial occupational disability even in the absence of any other psychological, psychiatric or organic brain disorder. Alcoholism is obviously not just a symptom, although it does frequently coexist with other psychiatric illnesses. Major long-term studies in representative samples have clearly shown alcohol consumption at time T1 – and not neurotocism scales or other tests – to be the best predictor of consumption at time T2.

The Question of Personal Blame in the Law and in Insurance Practice

Switzerland's legal system operates from the principle that all adults are responsible for their own lives and may live as they wish. The law thus affords tremendous scope for personal choices, including choices to act irrationally. However, the situation is entirely different where insurance companies are concerned. Health policies cover alcoholism only if it has been diagnosed by a specialist. Moreover, alcoholism in itself does not entitle the sufferer to disability benefits. To quality for benefits under the state disability scheme one also has to have a mental illness or physical or mental disability. It goes without saying that this position is at variance with the definitions in ICD-10 and DSM-IV. What is more, it is at variance with the wealth of scientific evidence that has been accumulated on the association between unemployment and alcohol dependence.

Conclusions

(1) Alcohol dependents remain a socially stigmatised group.

(2) The status of alcohol dependence as a disease is increasingly being denied. It is vital that it retains this status.

(3) Alcohol dependents are doubly discriminated against: in the workplace and in insurance practice.

(4) Employment is vital to the process of recovering from dependence; restrictions on eligibility for disability benefits are in no way justifiable.

References

Catalano R, Dooley D, Wilson G, Hough R: Job loss and alcohol abuse: A test using data from the Epidemiologic Catchment Area Project. J Health Soc Behav 1993;34:215–225.
Claussen B, Aasland OF: The Alcohol Use Disorders Identification Test (AUDIT) in a routine health examination of long-term unemployed. Addiction 1993;88:363–368.

Dooley D, Catalano R, Hough R: Unemployment and alcohol disorder in 1910 and 1990: Drift versus social causation. J Occup Organizational Psychol 1992;65:277–290.

Fahrenkrug H: Alkohol: Laster oder Krankheit? Schweiz Apothekerztg 1992;20:593–595.

Foucault M: Histoire de la folie. Paris, 1961.

Frone MR, Windle M: Job dissatisfaction and substance use among employed high school students: The moderating influence of active and avoidant coping styles. Subst Use Misuse 1997;32:571–585.

Janlert U, Hammarström A: Alcohol consumption among unemployed youths: Results from a prospective study. Br J Addict 1992;87:703–714.

Jellinek EM: Drinkers and alcoholics in ancient Rome. J Stud Alcohol 1976;37:11.

Maffli E, Wacker HR, Mathey MC: 7-Jahreskatamnese von stationär behandelten Alkoholabhängigen in der deutschen Schweiz. Schweizerische Fachstelle für Alkohol- und andere Drogenprobleme, Forschungsbericht 26.

Mullahy J, Sindelar J: Life-cycle effects of alcoholism on education, earnings, and occupation. Enquiry 1989;26:272–282.

Richard Müller, Schweizerische Fachstelle für Alkohol- und andere Drogenprobleme,
Avenue Ruchonnet 14, Case postale 870, 1001 Lausanne (Switzerland)
Tel. +41 21 321 29 11, Fax +41 21 321 29 40, E-Mail prevention@sfa-ispa.ch

Author Index

Besson, J. 40
Biedert, E. 45

Fenton, B.T. 29

Ihde, T. 45

Knoch, H. 45

Ladewig, D. VII, 45, 49
Lieb, R. 7

Müller, R. 56
Müller-Spahn, F. VIII

Perkonigg, A. 7
Preisig, M. 29

Spanagel, R. 1
Stohler, R. 23

von Bardeleben, U. 45

Wittchen, H.-U. 7

Subject Index

Acamprosate, alcohol relapse prevention 45–48

Acquired immunodeficiency syndrome
mortality in drug users 30
needle distribution in prevention 51

Adolescents, predictors of drug use and abuse 18–20

Adrenalectomy, effects on ethanol drinking in rats 1, 2

Alcohol
abstinence rates by sex and age 57, 58
adrenalectomy, effects on ethanol drinking in rats 1, 2
blame vs illness concept of alcoholism 57–62
comorbidity
drug disorders 30, 32, 33
psychiatric disorders 30, 31, 33, 34
study design 32, 35, 36
corticotropin-releasing hormone receptor, ethanol exposure and withdrawal in knockout mice 4, 5
history of dependence sociology 56, 57
legal and insurance implications of alcoholism 62
lifetime prevalence of abuse or dependence 29
psychoscience meshing with neuroscience in dependency 43
relapse prevention
acamprosate 45–48
disulfiram 45–48

naltrexone 45–48
psychotherapy 45–48, 52
risk factors for dependency 50, 51, 54
unemployment relationship to alcoholism
ability to work as a medical category 61, 62
discrimination in employment 60, 61
drift hypothesis 59, 60
social causation hypothesis 59, 60

Amphetamines
coabuse with other drugs 14, 15
lifetime prevalence of DSM-IV abuse or dependence 13, 14

Benzodiazepines, dependence 52, 53

Cannabis
coabuse with other drugs 14, 15, 19
drug interactions 52
lifetime prevalence of DSM-IV abuse or dependence 13, 14
patterns of use and abuse 15–20

Cocaine
coabuse with other drugs 14, 15
lifetime prevalence of DSM-IV abuse or dependence 13, 14
mood disorder comorbidity in users 31
pharmacotherapeutic intervention 52

Corticosterone, effects on ethanol drinking in rats 1, 2

Corticotropin-releasing hormone receptor,
   ethanol exposure and withdrawal in
   knockout mice 4, 5

Dependence, definition 49, 50
Diagnosis, clinical dependency research
   subjects 41, 49, 50
Disulfiram, alcohol relapse prevention
   45–48

Early Developmental Stages of
   Psychopathology study
   design and aims 10, 11
   findings
      baseline study 12–15
      follow-up study 15–18
      statistical analysis of risk factors
         18, 19
   methods 11, 12
   modeling theory 9, 10
Employment, see Unemployment
Epilepsy, heroin users
   anticonvulsant therapy 26, 28
   brain oxygenation in users 24–26
   electroencephalography studies
      24, 53
   psychosocial consequences 26, 28
Ethanol, see Alcohol

Glucocorticoid receptor
   antidepressant effects on expression
      4
   hypothalamic-pituitary-adrenocortical
      system regulation 2, 3
   morphine effects in antisense transgenic
      mice 2–4

Hallucinogens
   coabuse with other drugs 14, 15
   lifetime prevalence of DSM-IV abuse or
      dependence 13, 14
Heroin
   brain oxygenation in users 24–26
   electroencephalography studies 24, 53
   Janus Project 23
   pharmacokinetics 23, 24
   psychosocial consequences 26, 28

Hypothalamic-pituitary-adrenocortical
   system
   addiction role 1–6
   antidepressant effects on activity 4
   corticotropin-releasing hormone receptor,
      ethanol exposure and withdrawal in
      knockout mice 4, 5
   glucocorticoid receptor regulation
      2–4

Intervention, clinical dependency research
   subjects 41, 42

Longitudinal studies, addiction
   assessment instruments 9
   design 8
   multivariate modeling 18–20
   sampling 7, 8

Methadone, psychoscience meshing with
   neuroscience in treatment 44
Moclobemide, effects on glucocorticoid
   receptor expression 4
Mortality, drug-related mortality in
   Switzerland 29, 30

Naltrexone, alcohol relapse prevention
   45–48
Neuroscience vs psychoscience 40, 41
Nicotine, depression following withdrawal
   49

Opioids, see also Heroin
   coabuse with other drugs 14, 15
   lifetime prevalence of DSM-IV abuse or
      dependence 13, 14
   mood disorder comorbidity in users
      31
   mortality rate in users 30
   pharmacotherapeutic intervention 53
   side effects 53

Psychiatric disorders, comorbidity with
   drug use
   mechanisms
      alcoholism
         anxiety disorder 34

mood disorder 33, 34
   drugs with mood and anxiety
     disorders 35
   study design 32, 35, 36
  overview 30–32
Psychoscience vs neuroscience 40, 41
Psychotherapy, alcohol relapse prevention
  45–48, 52

Relapse prevention, *see* Alcohol

St. Martin Center, features 42, 43
Sampling, longitudinal studies of
  addiction 7, 8

Unemployment, relationship to alcoholism
  ability to work as a medical category
    61, 62
  discrimination in employment 60, 61
  drift hypothesis 59, 60
  social causation hypothesis 59, 60